Death Only Needs To
Win Once

Death Only Needs To Win Once

✦

The trials and tribulations of one Liverpool lad

William Carroll

iUniverse, Inc.
New York Bloomington Shanghai

Death Only Needs To Win Once
The trials and tribulations of one Liverpool lad

iUniverse books may be ordered through booksellers or by contacting:

iUniverse
1663 Liberty Drive
Bloomington, IN 47403
www.iuniverse.com
1-800-Authors (1-800-288-4677)

Because of the dynamic nature of the Internet, any Web addresses
or links contained in this book may have changed
since publication and may no longer be valid.

The views expressed in this work are solely those of the author and do
not necessarily reflect the views of the publisher, and the publisher
hereby disclaims any responsibility for them.

ISBN: 978-0-595-49844-4 (pbk)
ISBN: 978-0-595-61272-7 (ebk)

Printed in the United States of America

DEATH ONLY NEEDS TO WIN ONCE!

This book is dedicated to the memory of

LILIAN

My wife, My friend, My soulmate

FOREWORD

By rights I should have been dead a long time ago! So many things have happened to me over the years that could have culminated in my death, I should have been a goner many moons since. It makes me think that, like our feline friends, I must have nine lives, or maybe even more. The circumstances surrounding all the occasions that might have resulted in my dying have been varied and unusual to say the least.

In the pages ahead I will relate some of my life history, [mostly about my early years, when most of the dangerous situations happened] during which I will attempt to explain how each of these events evolved and how I ended up still here today. At the time of writing this, my age is 72 and it seems that it all started to go "RIGHT" from the age of 2 years.

There have been many books written about the pre World War 2 years and the war years themselves. This particular narrative is focused on some of the many problems which I myself encountered, during those years and beyond, along with some background information, and hence, it might not be as lengthy as some other renderings about that period. I hope the reader, after reading my story, will have a fair idea of some of the difficulties and dangers we faced as kids growing up in England during that era, although my story reaches far beyond my early days and into my retirement years.

Of the <u>seven</u> occasions when I consider that I had my lucky escapes from death, four of them happened by the time I was ten years old, one when I was sixteen, and the other two much later, during adulthood, while we were living in Canada, the latter of which happened when I was 65 years of age, [while on holiday in England].

In putting this story together I have been working from memory alone as there is nothing written down, particularly from my younger years, to clarify the details. I have had some help from my brother Charlie, as he is two years older than I, and he was able to remember more details than I could. Also, my elder sister Betty has been able to fill in some gaps for me. For this I thank them both.

1

We were a poor working class family, living in squalid conditions in down town Liverpool, England in the 1930's. I was born on 13th March 1935, and had a brother who was two years older, a sister who was 7, and of course my mother and father. The house we lived in was somewhat run-down and as we were a rather poor family we couldn't have afforded most of the amenities that most people take for granted today, even if they had been available in those days. There was an infestation of cockroaches in most houses in each street and the district itself had lots of rats in the area. Whenever we came home after dark and the gas light in the living room was lit, the cockroaches could be seen scurrying off to the darker corners of the room. As our coal supply was kept under the stairs, it should not be too surprising that they seemed to make their 'home' there. It was just something that we had to live with and accept.

Instead of a stove, all we had was a gas ring which sat upon our kitchen table. It was on this that we had to do most of our cooking. Our only source of heat in the house was a coal fireplace in the living room. Of course, there was an oven next to the fireplace which got it's heat from the fire. Some baking etc. could be done in this oven. For lighting, there was only the gas light in the ceiling of the living room, complete with a gas mantle. At bedtime we would have to carry a lighted candle [usually on a saucer] to see our way upstairs, and so that we could have some light up there.

Outside, at the rear of the house, there was a back yard which had an out-house containing a toilet. In the winter months a lighted candle would have to be left in there in an attempt to stop the pipes from freezing, even though the pipes were heavily lagged. Attached to the outside wall of the outhouse there was a big sink which had just a cold water tap. This tap was the only source of water for our household. [Provided through 'lead' piping] Times were very hard in those days and money was not easy to come by. My father used to get temporary work whenever possible, and we could barely eke out an existence. Should there be a spell of no work, there was always a miserly money lender who lived nearby who would lend families the princely sum of five shillings, which had to be repaid at tuppence [two pence] per week for about a year or so. If a loan of five shillings was paid back for 52 weeks at that rate, the interest for the year would have amounted to just over 73%, so you can see how money-lenders got rich off the backs of the poor, [Reminds me of Scrooge].

This was the sort of background of our existence during the pre World War 2 years and there were many families living in these sorts of conditions in downtown Liverpool during that period.

I was just two years old, when, one day my mother had a pan of water heating on the gas ring on the kitchen table, probably to make a pot of tea. As inquisitive kids do, I had to reach up to find out if I could see what was in the pan. I managed somehow to pull the pan off the gas ring, which caused the pan to tip over. The entire contents, which was now <u>boiling water,</u> emptied out and onto the top of my head.

The memory of that incident is imprinted on my brain, but what happened after that I cannot recall. I understand that I was rushed to the hospital, probably being carried in the old pram which had been used for me when I was a baby. The old Royal Hospital was approximately ten or fifteen minutes walk from where we lived. Of course nobody had telephones in those times, nor did anyone have a car. So we had to make our own way to the Hospital or to a doctor, either by using the tram-car or by walking. If there had been any such thing as a taxi available, we could not have afforded it any way.

In an emergency like this one, we were lucky to have been as close to the Hospital as we were; otherwise I might have died from the shock before help could be reached. What I do remember is that after my initial visit and treatment, I had to be taken to the out patient's clinic every day [walking of course] for about six weeks for the dressing on my head to be changed. The severe scalding had caused me to lose all the hair on my head and my scalp was just one big scab. There were two different treatments which I had on alternate days. One was from a bottle of clear liquid (probably an alcoholic base of some kind) which really stung my head and made me cry, while the other one was from a jar of a yellow coloured ointment which was very soothing and cool to my head. Each day as we walked to the Hospital, I used to say to my mother "Tell them I don't want the bottle, I want the egg." The yellow ointment must have reminded me of egg yolks.

After my head had fully healed, all my hair grew back. The doctor who had been treating me was most surprised to see that I had regained my hair, because, originally he thought that it would not grow back because of the severity of the injury. It had also retained its black colour and as it happens I still have a good head of hair today [age 72], but it is now white in colour. I was also lucky that I had not sustained any damage to my eyes.

As it was possible that I could have died from the shock, I consider this incident to have been my <u>first</u> lucky escape from death.

It was almost a year later that we were [UN] fortunate enough to qualify for a Corporation flat [property owned by the city, and rented out to needy families.] The property was located about three miles further out from town, in the district of Old Swan and consisted of several blocks of flats, which were commonly known as tenements, and our family was one of the first to move in. As I was only 3 years old at the time, I wasn't aware of any furniture being moved up from town to this new location. What I was told in later years was that everything we needed from the old house had to be trundled along on borrowed hand carts, which was quite a struggle, as most of the journey to Old Swan was uphill. We could not have afforded a moving van in those days and the goods had to be moved by family members or close relatives, and would have taken a few days to complete.

This new accommodation was considered, by us, to be a luxury residence, compared with the old house which we had left behind. There was a proper bathroom which contained a tub with hot and cold taps, a sink also with hot and cold taps and a toilet. In the living room there was a coal fireplace which had an oven alongside. We used to heat up clean house bricks in this oven and wrap them in a towel or pillowcase and take them to bed as makeshift hot water bottles, particularly in the winter. At the back of the fireplace there were some water pipes which, when heated by the fire, would supply hot water to a hot water storage tank in the kitchen, just off the living room. I recall that during the winter months the fire would be loaded up and packed with damp slack [coal dust] to keep the fire 'simmering' all night, so that there would still be hot water in the storage tank the following morning to enable us to get washed without having to boil a kettle of water. None of the properties had a shower installed which meant that one had to wash at the sink, either in the bathroom or the kitchen! Most people used to have a weekly bath. All the pipes in the flat were made of copper.

Of course, this also meant that the living room would still have some warmth in the morning, which made things a little more pleasant, especially in the winter months, and the fire would be kept going for the rest of the day, only to be 'packed up' again for the following night. The kitchen also had a gas stove, which was a tremendous upgrade from our old gas ring, and a pantry with ample food storage shelves and a cold marble slab for keeping food cool. However, we couldn't keep any meats or other perishables for very long, even on this marble slab. This is why families had to shop every day for such items and use them up the same day. [We didn't have the luxury of a refrigerator in those days]. I can recall that during the heat of summer we had to immerse our bottles of milk in a sink filled with cold water and hope this would stop it from going sour overnight. As old habits die hard, one can still find many of the older people doing their daily shopping, in spite of now having the convenience of refrigerators. Of course, as each new generation comes along, shopping is done less frequently and deep freezers are now widely used in most homes. There was also a sink in the kitchen which had hot and cold taps, and a gas boiler for washing clothes which had a mangle attached for wringing out the washing.

The flat contained three bedrooms, two of which had fireplaces, which were often used during the winter months. [What we would have given for a central heating system]. As these blocks of flats were new buildings, they obviously had electricity throughout and we thought it was fantastic to just flick a switch to have the room lit up. Overall, this new place was a definite luxury after the conditions we had to endure in our previous house. At this time my mother was expecting another baby which eventually turned out to be my younger sister. I remember my mother was scolding me for something one day [I don't remember what for] and I ran away from her and cheekily shouted back at her "fat belly". She was pretty heavy 'with child' at the time, but my being only three years old, I didn't know why she was 'fat'. This caused my mother to laugh. [Dare I say a good 'belly laugh'?]

Another good thing about this modern flat was that there was no infestation of cockroaches, nor were there any rats in the area. But a few years later we had a plague of fleas from the field which was at the back of our tenements. Our flats were being overrun by them and I remember that as young kids we wore short trousers, and as soon as we walked into the flat, the fleas were all over our legs. We attacked them with lots of D.D.T. [which is banned from use nowadays,] and we eventually managed to get rid of them. But it was no fun while the battle was going on. While this situation continued we couldn't bring any friends over, as it would have been too embarrassing, although those of my friends who lived in the same tenements were undergoing a similar problem at their flats. One could imagine how horrible it would have been to have one's friends or relatives 'attacked' by a swarm of those fleas.

I recently learned a very interesting fact about fleas. Apparently, they are reputed to be able to jump to about 130 times their own height. This would be the equivalent of a 6 ft. person jumping to a height of 780 ft. Now, THAT would be some kind of high jump record wouldn't it?

2

When the Second World War started in September 1939 we were still living in the flat in Liverpool England and I was four and a half years old. I had just started school, and I can remember the first day when my mother took me there. I was left in the infants class for that first morning and there was a 'large' rocking horse in the classroom upon which I was placed by the teacher and some of the other kids started to rock me [in my opinion] so violently, that I thought I was going to be thrown off. I just hung on 'for grim death'. The next thing I recall was my mother coming to collect me and take me home at lunchtime. After lunch we headed back towards the school, and I asked my mother "Do I have to go again?" Little did I know how many more 'agains' there were going to be throughout the next several years.

During World War 2, certain strategic locations across Great Britain were bound to be targeted by the bombing raids from Germany, such as major ports and airports. Liverpool had seven miles of docklands, as well as an Airport. There was also a Power Station that was only about a half mile from where we lived. Because of the dangers that were expected to follow the declaration of war, the government started a campaign to 'save the children'. This meant that as many children as possible would be sent to live in the countryside, well away from any areas that could be devastated by multiple bombing raids. This was known as 'EVACUATION'. Children would only be evacuated with their parents consent and they could possibly remain away from home until the war ended. This campaign was going on all over Britain and there were many thousands of children sent away to presumably safer havens under this scheme.

My father had already joined the army and had been posted to a camp somewhere, presumably to train in readiness for the conflict that was bound to start at any time. Myself [Billy] aged 4, my brother [Charlie] aged 6, and our elder sister [Betty], aged 11, were all to be evacuated, whilst our new baby sister [Joan], then aged 1 year, was to remain at home in Liverpool with our mother.

The designated day arrived, when we were to be transported, by bus, to various locations in North Wales. All the children had name tags attached to their coats, and we all had gas masks, in their cases, slung over our shoulders. My brother Charlie and I spent a short time billeted at Llangollen, and also at a place called Tyn-y-coed. Eventually, we arrived at our final destination, which was a little town called Llandudno Junction. This was just across the Conway River from the popular tourist town of Conway, which sported Conway Castle that was strategically placed at the end of the Conway Bridge. This location was approximately 100 miles from Liverpool and was considered to be at a safe enough distance from any possible conflict. Our sister Betty had been dropped off at a little town called Abergele and that was the last we saw of her until we were all back in Liverpool.

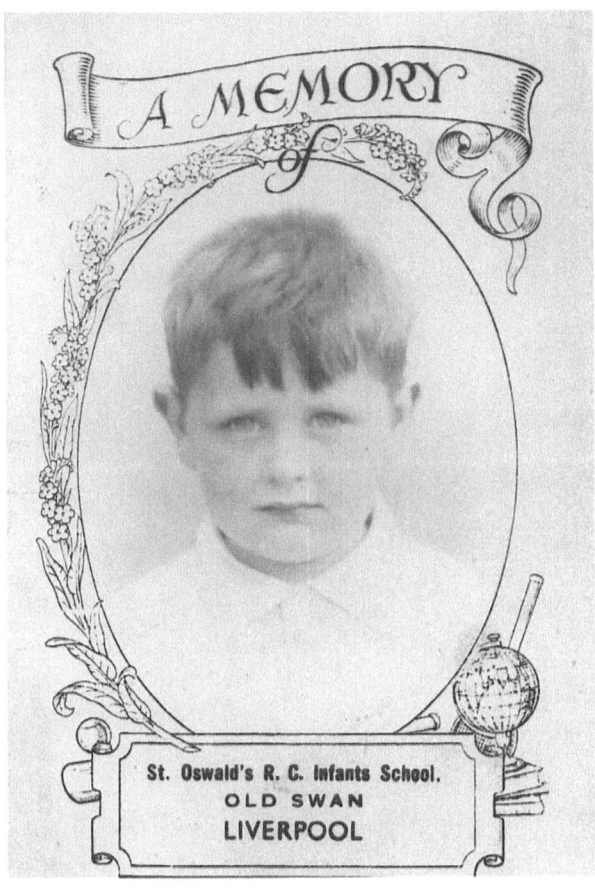

St. Oswald's R. C. Infants School,
OLD SWAN
LIVERPOOL

This is a picture of me [William Carroll] which was taken just after I had started school at the age of four. Unfortunately, I cannot find any other pictures of me from around that period.

This would be what I looked like at the time that we were evacuated to North Wales in September 1939.

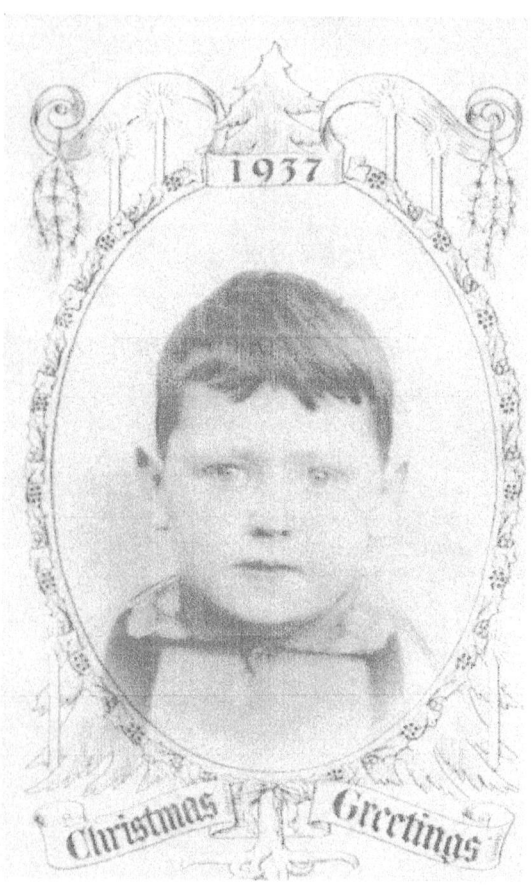

This is a photo of my brother Charlie, taken when he was just four years old. It is the only picture of him from around that period. It was two years after this was taken that we were evacuated to North Wales at the start of World War 2.

The accommodations seemed to have all been pre-allotted and my brother and I, along with six other young boys, were billeted in a big house, [called Cornerways] which had been converted into a virtual boarding house. A large bedroom had been arranged with 8 single beds, [four along one wall and four along the wall opposite] sort of barrack style. We were each given our own single bed.

In later years Charlie adopted the name 'Cornerways' for his own house, in Sutton-on-Forest, near York, as a memento of those years of long ago.

The owner of the house was an older lady who treated all the boys very well and we all liked her, and got along very nicely with her.

As I had already started school in Liverpool [which was normal at age four in Britain at that time] I was required to attend school, along with my brother Charlie, although, he would be in a separate class as he was two years older. All the boys were assigned to local schools according to their religious backgrounds and as our background was Catholic, we were sent to the nearest Catholic school, which happened to be across the bridge in Conway. I remember that the approach road to the castle was separated from what was known as the Cobb by a low wall which had gaps in it. Some of the gaps were narrow and some of them were wide. As we were going to and from school, we would walk along on the wall and jump across the gaps as we went. When we were approaching the wider gaps [which were about six feet wide] we would have to take a run at them so that we could leap across them. When we visited the area many years later as adults, I could not believe that a four year old could actually leap across those wider gaps. I don't think I could have done so as an adult, but I know I really did manage to do it when I was four years old. We used to come home at lunch time and return to school in the afternoon. This meant that we had to walk across the 'famous' Conway Bridge four times a day. There was, in those days, an actual walkway attached to the side of the bridge, which we used. This walkway was removed several years later as it was considered unsafe, because of it's vast age. Incidentally, many more years later the bridge was given a total overhaul which included the scraping off of all the layers of old paint. I understand that the total weight of all the old paint that was scraped off amounted to over 300 tons.

At about the same time as the walkway was removed, a new road bridge was built, including a sidewalk, parallel to the old iron bridge, which was then closed to traffic and the old bridge then became just another tourist attraction.

Conway was always a bad bottleneck for traffic, and remained so, even with the new road bridge, but it was many years later that, to alleviate this forever increasing problem, a road tunnel was built re-directing 'through' traffic under the Conway river, to by-pass the town altogether. It certainly improved the traffic flow, in both directions, which was headed to all the other North Wales resorts.

Whilst we were attending the school at Conway, there were a couple of unusual incidents that I was involved in, that were quite dangerous. Myself and another boy in my class both had a loose tooth and we were competing with each other to see who would be the first to get his tooth out. We were both jiggling our teeth back and forth, when I had a 'brilliant' idea. I just punched myself in the mouth and out came my tooth. So, I guess I won, but the only prize I got was a bleeding lip, to add to my bleeding gum. As we had not heard of the tooth fairy in those days we did not receive any monetary exchange for our teeth and they were just thrown away. [Sad].

The other incident that occurred, involved a further competition with another boy, to see who could cram the most marbles into his mouth. We were both shoving the marbles in pretty quickly, when, suddenly, I swallowed one of mine. The teacher was told and right away she sent for an ambulance. I was taken to the hospital and I can remember lying on a bed, or a table and the doctor had an oblong screen over me, which I now presume to have been an x-ray machine. Someone pointed at something and said "Is that it there?" and somebody else answered, "No, that's a button on the back of his pants". We used to have buttons on our pants to fasten our braces to, [In North America they would be known as suspenders.]

I don't know if the offending marble was ever located or not, but I suppose, as it was made of glass, it would be difficult to see. One can only assume that it passed right through my system and out, but I don't recall anything else being done about it. There was the possibility that it could have caused internal problems, but I didn't seem to suffer any further difficulties in the weeks following. I was also lucky enough not to have choked on that marble.

Another incident which comes to mind was when we were playing in Conway while on the way home. We were running in and out of the Woolworths store, which had doors that swung back and forth past each other. I was holding on to one of the doors when the other one swung past splitting the end of my thumb. It bled profusely and I recall a policeman taking me into the police station for first aid treatment. It was very sore when he held it under the cold water tap before bandaging it up. I still have a scar on that thumb today and it always reminds me of how it happened.

It's amazing what sorts of stupid things most young kids get up to sometimes.

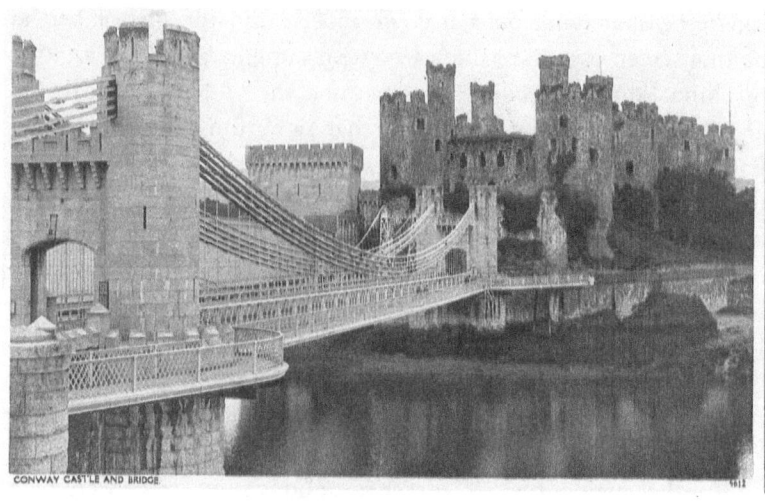

CONWAY CASTLE AND BRIDGE

Conway Bridge as it was in 1939 showing the walkway, along its side, which my brother Charlie and I used to cross the bridge on our way to and from School in Conway.

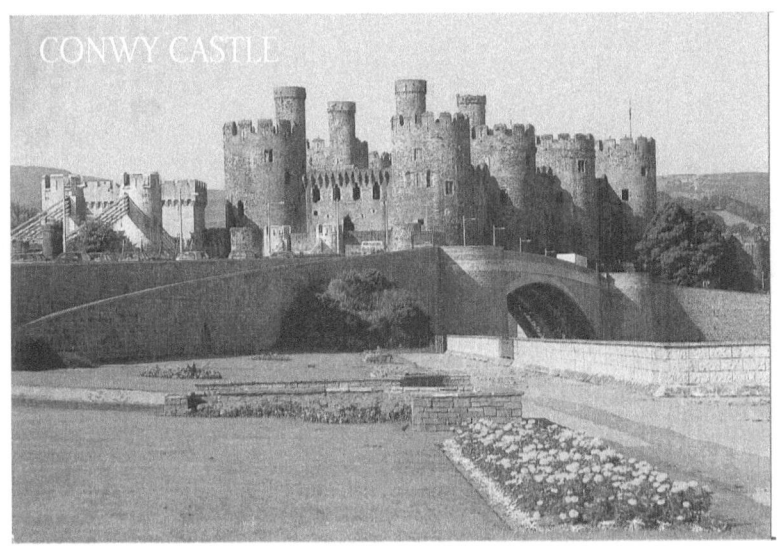

A picture postcard of Conway Castle in the 1990's showing the old Bridge partly obscured by the new Road Bridge. In the forefront is a section of the "Cobb" referred to earlier in the book. One can see how the castle has been refurbished.

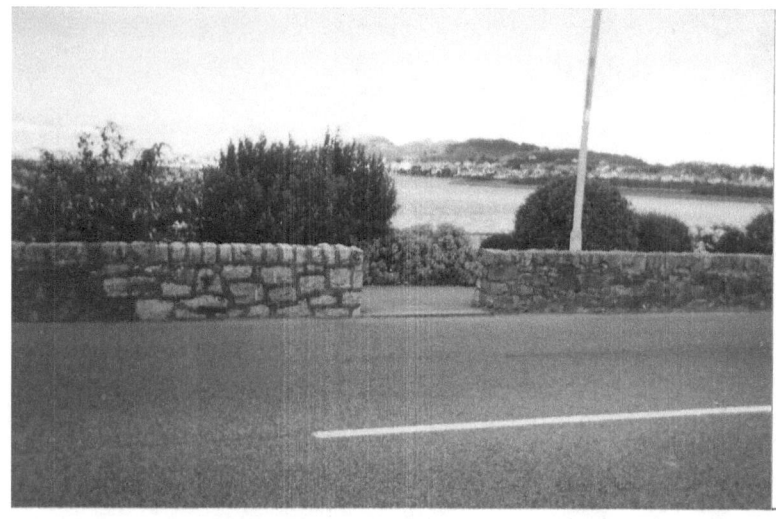

The wall separating the approach road to Conway Bridge, from the Cobb, showing one of the larger gaps in it which we used to jump [leap] across, successfully, when I was only 4 and 5 years old.

3

Whenever we were allowed out to play, at our evacuation digs, we mostly went to a local park, which was just a few blocks away. There were some swings there, as well as a pond and also some bushes and trees at one side of the park. One particular day my brother Charlie and I decided to play by the pond, which was surrounded by a small wall about one foot high. We had never actually been in the water in the pond, so we did not know how deep it was, and anyway it seemed too dirty to venture into it, as it was somewhat stagnated. On this day, when the other boys were either playing on the swings or in among the bushes, Charlie and I were playing at the pond's edge. I had fashioned a small 'boat' out of a matchbox and was 'sailing' it [pushing it along with my hand; It is amazing what a four year old's imagination can come up with.] However, my 'boat' started to float away from the edge, and I was reaching out for it, to bring it back, leaning out over the little wall. Suddenly, I had overreached myself and I overbalanced and went tumbling literally 'head over heels' into the murky water.

I cannot remember all that happened after that, but what I do recall, from all those years ago, was, sitting upright at the bottom of the pond, with the water well above my head. I noticed a little beetle swimming past in front of my face and I just sat there completely disorientated, with no idea of what was happening. If my brother had not been there and done something to get me out, I most certainly would have just sat there and drowned. I believe, from his recollection of the occasion, that he reached into the pond and pulled me up out of the water by grabbing me by the hair. He then gave me a piggyback home. Thank goodness I regained all my hair after losing it all when I was two years old, from that severe scalding. This near drowning was what I consider to be my <u>second</u> lucky escape from the jaws of death. If I had been playing on my own at that time, I certainly would not have survived.

It was some weeks later that my next brush with death occurred. We were enjoying a nice spring day, warm and sunny with plenty of fluffy white clouds floating along in the sky. We were happily playing in a wooded area, having an adventure, pretending we were Robin Hood and his merry men. Somehow I had wandered off the edge of the path which ran through the woods. I must have disturbed a bees' hive, as they sometimes make their hives in the ground. All of a sudden I found myself covered by a swarm of angry bees, and I was being stung all over every exposed part of me. At that age [I was just 5 years old at that time] I wore short pants and a short sleeved shirt, so the bees had plenty of target area to attack, including my face and neck. I must have had well over a hundred stings, complete with lumps, and enough venom in me to kill an elephant. I can remember the incident quite well, but I cannot recall how I managed to get away from them, nor how I got home. Once again I think that I was rescued by my brother Charlie. I don't even know if I was treated by a doctor or taken to a hospital, or how long it took for all the lumps to go down. A person who had an allergy to bee stings would most certainly have died from an attack of this magnitude, but even so, with the amount of venom I must have had in me, I was very lucky not to have succumbed to it myself. I feel that this incident could well have resulted in my death, and that is why I consider that this was my <u>third</u> lucky escape from death's clutches.

As I mentioned earlier, all the boys at our billet got on very well with the lady who owned the house and we were all treated more or less like family. We were all enjoying staying there, but things were about to change somewhat. I am not sure for how long we had enjoyed this pleasant state of affairs, but the house was about to change hands and things would not be the same anymore. In fact they would become rather unpleasant compared with the nice time we had been having.

The new owner was an officer in the Home Guard and was married with one young son. This new family took up residence and whereas, before, all of the boys had had free run of the whole house [just like any normal family] the new owners made certain areas of the house out of bounds to us. A section of the house was to be for him and his family only. As most military officers do, this one also carried a swagger stick [an army cane.] We, [meaning all of the evacuees at this house] came to 'know' this swagger stick, only too well, in the months that followed. Whenever any of the boys was found to be doing something that he shouldn't, the owner would keep a note of the incident, and once per week, in true military style, he would hold a 'court martial' and any miscreants would have punishment meted out to them for their misdemeanors, despite the fact that we were all young children. We would all be seated around the large dining table which was used for the 'court martial', and as each 'culprit's' name was read out, he would have to go to the end of the table, where our 'commanding officer' would be seated. The offender would have his pants taken down and he would be bent over the end of the table and be caned across the bare buttocks with the swagger stick. The number of strokes he received was according to the owner's idea of the severity of the 'offence'. In my own particular case I can remember one occasion when I was 'punished' in this way because I had had a little accident and had marked my underwear. The fact that I was only just five years old didn't seem to matter. Such child abuse would not be tolerated this day and age. In fact an abuser such as this would probably be sent to prison.

Because of all the abuse, my brother Charlie and another boy from his class at school that he had befriended, who was also an evacuee, decided to run away. Of course they were both only seven years old and had vivid imaginations. They had equipped themselves with a small amount of food and some water and were going to make their way along the road to Bangor which was several miles away. After a few miles the other boy lost his nerve and turned back. Charlie had decided to continue all by himself. I am not certain how long it took for his absence to be noticed, but apparently there were police looking for him. His objective was to steal a rowing boat when he reached Bangor and row to India, where our father was purported to be stationed in the army. When you look at the World map, India does not look too far away so Charlie's plan didn't seem that bad to him. He was, of course, subsequently picked up by the police and apparently his little escapade made headlines in a local Newspaper.

When Charlie and I were both visiting Conway [on a 'memory lane' trip] in 2005, both of us in our seventies, we tried to find a copy of the paper which ran the story but we did not know the specific dates nor the name of the actual newspaper. Hence, our search was to no avail. I am sure it must be somewhere in the paper's archives. It would be really something special to have a copy of that story to show to family and friends. Of course, as soon as our Mother heard of Charlie's running away and also the abuse we were being subjected to, she made arrangements for both of us to be brought back home to Liverpool, despite the fact that the war was still going on, and Liverpool was still being bombed, almost nightly, by the German Luftwaffe.

4

When we arrived back in Liverpool we found it to be quite different from when we left it, especially in the hours after dark. There were no street lights allowed nor any lights coming from residences, or businesses. Everyone had been informed that a state of 'BLACK-OUT' was to be observed after dark. Every window was to be covered with either a black cloth, or some other opaque material, so that there were no lights showing. This was to prevent any lights being seen by enemy aircraft which might give them something to aim at. Air-raid Wardens were patrolling the streets to see that everyone was conforming, and if any shaft of light was showing, a warden would draw the occupier's attention to it and the light would be covered up.

When any enemy aircraft had been observed to be heading in our general direction, air-raid sirens would blare out their ominous warnings and then everyone would proceed to their appointed air-raid shelter. These shelters, of which there had been hundreds built around the city, mainly in the residential areas, were fairly solid brick structures which had a concrete slab roof, usually one storey high, with no windows, just air vents, and an offset doorway at either end, so that no direct light could be seen coming from inside the shelter. Inside there was very dim lighting and bunk beds had been installed along one side. Families in the near vicinity had particular spaces assigned to them, although anyone in need was welcome. The bunk beds had straw mattresses and we provided our own blankets. These beds were very handy for younger children as they afforded them somewhere to sleep, because on most nights we were closeted in the shelters for many hours until the enemy aircraft had left the area and the sirens had sounded the 'all clear'. We used to hate hearing the sirens going off, but it seemed to happen almost every night. The loud speakers, through which the sound was transmitted, were strategically located around the area and were positioned high up on poles so that their sound could be easily heard. When they did 'blast off', we went through a routine of collecting our 'readied' bundles of blankets, snacks, drinks, candles, [for extra light if we might want to read], some reading matter, and torches [flash lights] to light our bleary eyed way to the shelter.

The shelters were to protect the people from any blast and/or flying debris, should any bombs fall in the near vicinity. However, if a bomb had made a direct hit on one, there would probably be many occupants killed, as these shelters were not bomb-proof.

It was only a few weeks after we had returned to Liverpool that a road only about one hundred yards from us, as the crow flies, namely Pemberton Road, was flattened by what we believed was a land mine intended to hit the Power Station that was approximately a half mile away from were we lived. The aircraft, which had missed it's target, had also made a strafing run at the Power Station, and there were big shell holes along the concrete wall which bordered it. That wall, with all it's tell tale historical shell markings, was left there for many years after the war had ended but has since been removed. I am not sure whether or not some part of it was kept showing the scars of warfare, but if it was up to me, a section of that wall would be in a military museum.

One particular night, after the sirens had sounded their foreboding warnings, we were making our almost nightly pilgrimage to the shelter complete with the usual bundles, and I decided to look up at the night sky, which happened to be clear that night. I was just trying to follow the light beam from the search light, when I noticed that several search lights from different areas had converged and were illuminating several airplanes [presumably enemy ones] and were tracking them across the sky. The noise was almost deafening as anti-aircraft guns from all over were constantly firing at them. Usually the guns were silent most nights as there were no visible targets to fire at. So this night was different with lots of noise, as the soldiers went about their business with lots of fervour. I can still remember the horrible droning sound of those planes. [I think they were Dorniers]. As kids would, we thought it was great to see and hear all this, but of course, we did not consider the damage that the plane's pay load was going to inflict on Liverpool, nor the devastation that might ensue, should a plane be shot down, before completing it's mission, and a whole plane load of bombs happened to crash into a residential area. The resultant explosion would be tremendous, with all the bombs going off at the same time, and many peoples lives could be lost in such a situation. But then again, it was wartime, and this is how it was. Those planes had to be stopped, at any cost, if at all possible, as the many miles of Liverpool's dockland was so vulnerable and had an extremely important role to play. Thousands of tons of supplies, and armaments needed by the Allied Forces, and civilians, were being shipped into Liverpool's docks continually, and they were being forwarded to the appropriate destinations as quickly as possible. There was not much sleeping going on that night in any of the shelters in our area. Another thing which comes to mind is, if any kids did not turn up for school, we just assumed that they might have been killed in the bombing raids. There were no such things as counsellors in the schools and we just had to go about our normal routines, as such things were to be expected while the War was going on, and once again we took it in our stride. There was no knowing if any of us had suffered mentally or emotionally from all that was happening, but we all just had to get on with it. As we were only kids, we never considered that on any one night it might be our turn to get killed in one of the bombing raids.

As fortune [or possibly misfortune] would have it, it is one of those air-raid shelters which features in my next narrow escape from death, but before I get into that story I would like to relate to you some of the growing up period, prior to, and after the War's end and some of the dangers we put ourselves in, just by making up our own games, and using some of the 'toys' which we fashioned for ourselves.

During our pre teen years all the kids in the neighbourhood used to play in the street or in the nearby playground which had swings, roundabout, monkey bars, etc. When we had tired of playing there we would go off to the park, about a mile away, or to Woolton woods which was about three miles away. Everywhere we went we used to walk, as we did not have money for trams or buses. If we did have any coppers [low valued coins] they would be held onto until we needed some money to purchase supplies for making any toys etc. The amount of energy we put out each day, with all our activities, ensured that we didn't put on much fat. Obese kids were few and far between in those days. Also, the fact that food was rationed helped to keep us slim. I can remember the long food lines whenever any fruit arrived at the greengrocer's, or any bread deliveries arrived at the bread shop.

We were not lucky enough to have all kinds of toys and gadgets or electronic games like most kids seem to have nowadays, so we used to make our own 'toys'. I remember using a penknife to cut off a small branch from a tree to make a bow, [as in bows and arrows]. It is amazing how skillful one can be when one has to be. The penknife was used to clean off the branch by cutting off all the small shoots or knots until the 'stick' was completely smooth. It also had to be tested to see if there was enough spring in it after it was bent into the bow shape. When it was acceptable, two notches would be cut in it, one at each end, to accommodate the string or twine, [which we always seemed to have enough of]. This would be knotted at one end to fit into one of the notches. The 'bow' was then bent to the required shape and the twine was pulled through the other notch until the 'bow' was just right, and it was held in place while the second knot was tied to complete the bow. Both ends of the bow were then bound tightly to stop them from splitting. We became so adept at this that I am sure Robin Hood would have been proud to have us in his band [of merry men].

When it came to 'arrows', we could purchase canes, [with the few pennies we could scrape together] from a local flower shop, which were about 2 foot 6 inches long and were most suitable for the purpose. The summers always seemed to be long and hot when we were kids, and the tarmac on the road surface was made soft by the heat. We would dig out some of the tarmac and stick it around the flower canes about three or four inches from one end. The 'arrows' worked very well when made this way, and we could literally fire them out of sight straight up in the air. They seemed to work just fine without any flights on the other ends, as the weighted ends could keep them flying straight. It was fortunate that none of us ever got hit by one of them falling back to earth. Serious damage could have been inflicted on a person should he have been hit on the head by one of them. We spent many hours having fun with our makeshift 'bows and arrows'.

During the winter months there was another 'dangerous' toy we used to make to occupy our time. We called it a 'winter warmer'. The requirements for this would consist of an empty tin can with the lid removed, a length of wire of about 3 to 4 feet, a large nail, a brick to use as a hammer to hit the nail, some newspaper, bits of wood for kindling, some small pieces of coal, [which was easy to come by as we all had coal fires at home], and of course some matches.

The can would be punctured, using the nail and brick, putting lots of holes under the base and around the sides, for ventilation, and two holes at the rim of the can, opposite each other, to accommodate the ends of the wire to enable us to form a long loop with the wire. The paper was placed in the bottom of the can followed by the kindling wood and the coal would be placed on top of the wood. The paper would be ignited, which in turn, would light the wood. We would swing the whole thing around in the air using the attached wire loop to get maximum air flow and eventually the coal would ignite and we would have our 'winter warmer', which was more or less just a miniature brazier. Once it was burning properly we would keep it topped up with coal and it would keep going for hours on end. [Of course we were employing several scientific principles without realising it.] Eventually it would be glowing red hot and when it was time to go in for the night we would have the problem of putting it out, only to start all over again the next night.

I previously referred to it as a 'dangerous' toy because I can recall one occasion when a boy was hit on the head by a 'winter warmer' that another boy was swinging around. He might have been severely burned by it as the contents spilled around him, but on this occasion he only seemed to suffer a lump on his head.

There were times in some winters when we couldn't get the pieces of coal we needed for our 'winter warmers' because there were often periods when coal was in short supply and our families would run out of coal altogether. It was so bad on occasions that we were reduced to burning anything suitable that we could find just to heat our homes. I remember when we were burning old shoes, pieces of linoleum, or any wood we could lay our hands on. Even old chairs would be broken up and burned. Believe me, things did get desperate sometimes.

As we were all dare devil kids in those times, we used to get up to all kinds of dangerous activities. Our blocks of flats [tenements that they were known as] were four storeys high and we would climb up the drain pipe on the top landing and onto the roof. We would play around up there, chasing each other, and sometimes run along on the parapet which ran along the edge of the roof, and was approximately 35 to 40 feet from the ground. We never gave any thought to the danger we might be in doing such things. If we had, we would never have enjoyed ourselves like we did.

Another particularly dangerous game that we played was 'war', using BB guns. One of my friends [Malcolm Grey] had two Webly pistols and an air rifle, while another boy had an air rifle, making four guns in all. Four of us would go to the park and split into two pairs and play war against each other. We were not experts with these guns but we used to have great fun with them. Most of the time nobody got hit, but I do remember once when I hit another lad on the bare arm which left him with a big bruise. Any one of us might well have been hit in the eye and possibly lost that eye, or maybe lost the sight in it, but with our devil-may-care attitude, we didn't give any thought to the possible dangers. We just enjoyed ourselves.

Another kind of 'war' game we played consisted of firing bent nails at each other. Somehow we would acquire a packet of small elastic bands and loop them together until we had a sufficient length to use as a catapult, using our thumb and first finger to loop the ends over. Believe me, this made an excellent catapult. We would search all over the place for nails to bend to use as ammunition. There were plenty of 'bombed out' houses around the area which contained lots of nails of various sizes and condition. Some of them were rusty but we used them anyway. The nails would be bent by using a brick and the curbside to knock them into the required shape, which was being bent double. Most of them would bend unevenly with the pointed end usually longer than the end with the head on it. As long as they had enough space between the ends so that they could be 'loaded' on to the elastics and fired, they were acceptable. One day while we were playing with them, I saw one of the 'enemy' boys get hit in the leg by one of the nails. It had hit him pointed end first and it had stuck in his calf. We all thought it was great that one of the 'enemy' had been wounded, but it didn't feel so good for him. At one point in the 'game' I had loaded a nail onto my elastic catapult and was taking careful aim, with one eye closed and the other one looking along the line of sight. When I released the nail, assuming it was headed for one of the 'enemy', the nail shot forward, but instead of heading for it's intended target, it just spun around on the elastic and came right back, hitting me in my eye. I was very lucky, because when the nail hit my eye, it struck me with the curved end and not the pointed end. Had it hit pointed end first I would have probably lost the sight in that eye. I know it was pretty painful at the time, but as luck would have it, there was no lasting damage, and to this day I still cannot remember which eye it was.

There was another very dangerous activity that we used to get up to when we wanted to go down town and we did not have any money for the tram fare. We would go up to the main road traffic lights and 'skip a lacker' [hang from the back of a suitable vehicle] and hang on for grim death until we reached our intended destination. We would wait until a suitable lorry would be stopped at the red light. When the light changed to green we would run out behind it [amidst all the traffic] and grab onto the tailgate and try to find something to rest our feet on, on the underside of the lorry, usually the spare tyre rack. This position would be maintained all the way to town, which was 3 to 4 miles. The biggest danger was the possibility that one of us might lose his grip and fall under the wheels of the following traffic, but it never did seem to happen. Mostly we would be heading for the dock road, along which there were many storage warehouses that always seemed busy either taking goods in or shipping goods out. We looked for a warehouse where they were using a simple rope hoist which was just looped around sacks to lift them to the level that they were to be stored at. Invariably, we found the right 'target' and after waiting patiently, [for as long as it took], a sack would slip out from the rope and plunge to the ground. When they hit the ground, the sacks usually burst open and the contents would be scattered around. This was our signal to jump in and grab whatever the cargo was, if it was worth having. The two most popular cargoes were peanuts and coconut shells, which still had the white lining inside. We would fill our pockets or bags, if we had any, and make ourselves scarce, before any of the workmen could stop us. I am not sure if it was true or not but someone told us that the coconuts were headed for the soap factory, but never the less, we enjoyed munching on them anyway.

When we had finished our scavenging activities, we would make our way home with the remainder of the spoils, [sounds like we were a bunch of pirates, but I would prefer the term 'salvagers']. We never did try to 'hitch' a ride back home. Maybe it was because we were still loaded up with our booty, so we could not hang on to the back of a lorry, without possibly dropping the goods. Hence it took a lot longer to get home than it did for us to get down town, but we were used to long treks. Circumstances being what they were in those days, we walked just about everywhere.

A somewhat humourous incident occurred one day when a few of us were at a loose end and we decided to rent some bicycles. About a mile or so down the road to town there was a man who used to fix up old bikes in his back yard and rent them out to kids in the area for sixpence an hour. So we decided, when we were 'flush', to go for a walk down to his yard where he operated from. There was one little problem. The kids who lived in our blocks of tenements had acquired somewhat of a reputation. They were regarded as a bunch of hooligans, and from this mans experience, he had had some of his bikes damaged by these kids. Hence, he would no longer rent his bikes to kids if he thought they were from these tenements. So, as we were walking along the main road I hit on a plan. There were only four of us at this particular time and I said to the others, "If he asks us where we live, tell him we come from this particular road" [which was only a few blocks from the man's yard]. The road's name was Onslow Road and I made sure we all had our story straight. We arrived at the yard a few minutes later and when we asked for the bikes he looked at us suspiciously and he said, "You kids are from those tenements, aren't you?" and, of course, we said that we were not. He then said, "Well, where do you live then?" One of the kids looked at me and said in a loud voice, "What's the name of that road?" [The stupid idiot]. The man obviously heard him and right away 'chucked' us out of his yard and we didn't get the bikes. At least we got the exercise of walking there and back.

When the War ended in June of 1945, I can remember all the celebrations that went on. Each street, well decorated with bunting, had a big party and every family provided all the necessary tables and chairs which were lined up along the whole length of each street. They also supplied all the cutlery [duly identified, usually by bits of string tied to each item so that the rightful owners would get them back when all the festivities were over] and there was an abundance of all kinds of foodstuffs both savoury and sweet. As children, we were only concerned with soft drinks, but I bet there were also plentiful supplies of alcoholic beverages for the adults. Anyway, a gay old time was had by all [if one can say that these days].

As mentioned previously in the chapter, my next brush with death involves one of the air-raid shelters. The war had ended some months earlier and all the shelters had had the doorways bricked up and were left where they stood for quite a while before eventually being demolished. People were beginning to rebuild their lives. Jobs were being created and food, although still rationed to the populace, was creeping back into the stores. I was now ten tears old. A neighbour of ours had a job driving a lorry [truck] which had an open flat-bed surrounded by sides and a tailgate which were about 18 inches high. It was this lorry along with an air-raid shelter that both feature in my next 'happening'. Mr. Taylor, who was the driver of the lorry, sometimes brought the lorry home at lunch time and when he was going back to work for the afternoon, he would often give the kids, who were around, a little treat by letting them all have a ride in the back of it. He would only take them to the top of the street, and then disembark them, before venturing out on to the main road. Part way up the street there was one of the now aban-doned air-raid shelters which had been built on the street, virtually blocking one half of the road surface. On one of these occasions, as the kids were all piling onto the back of the lorry, I was some dis-tance away and before I could get to it and climb aboard, Mr. Tay-lor had started off. Not wanting to miss my treat, I ran towards them, and as the route of the lorry took it around a playground, I ran across it to intercept them. I caught up with the lorry just as it had slowed down to make the turn onto the street which led to the main road. I managed to jump up and grab onto the side of the lorry but because of the impetus of the centrifugal force as it acceler-ated around the corner I could not climb onto the flatbed. The lorry sped up the road where it had to pass the shelter, and there was only about 6 or 8 inches clearance between them, and I was still hanging on to the side. It was just then that my brother Charlie, who hap-pened to be on board the lorry, reached over and grabbed my coat and pulled me over the side and on to the flatbed. One or two sec-onds later my body would have collided with the edge of the shelter and most probably, I would have sustained fatal injuries. The lorry was travelling at about 30 miles per hour [maybe even more]. I can-not see how I could have survived such an impact. Once again my brother had come to my rescue and most likely saved my life. If Charlie had not been on the lorry on that particular occasion, I do not think that any one of the other kids on board would have bothered to help me and it would have been "game over" for me. I reckon this event was definitely my <u>fourth</u> lucky escape from death. Of course Mr. Taylor did not know any of this was happening. I am sure that had he seen me running after the lorry he would have most likely stopped to let me on. As it turned out, my ride in the lorry was no fun at all. I was no sooner on it than I had to get off it again.

During the last three of my four narrow 'escapes' so far, my brother Charlie was instrumental in saving the day and I owe him a lot. Indeed I owe him my life [several times over]. While all these things were happening, we just did not appreciate how serious all these events really were. At the ages that we were, we just seemed to take everything in our stride. Here I was, still only ten years old and I had had what I believe to have been <u>four</u> lucky escapes from death.

There were several other occasions when I suffered various kinds of head trauma, none of which do I consider serious enough to be included in my list of narrow escapes from death, but still worthwhile mentioning, although I am rather vague about actual dates.

One time I was playing by myself, throwing a nice flat stone [the sort one would like to skim across the surface of water] straight up into the air, just to see if I could throw it out of sight. I do not think it actually went out of sight but it did go quite high up. I was watching it as it started to come back down and it seemed to be heading straight for me, so I stepped to one side so that it would not hit me. I thought I was out of line with it's trajectory when, because of it's nice flat shape, it swerved in the air and managed to hit me on the top of my head. It had made such a gash on my head that blood was pouring down my face and I ran home where my mother administered first aid and somehow stopped it from bleeding. It caused a rather big lump on my head which took several days to go down. I may have suffered a slight concussion but we did not worry about such things in those days. Of course I was out playing again as soon as my first aid was complete.

The monkey bars in the local playground, which was just yards away from our flat, were very useful for strengthening our arm and shoulder muscles as I am sure most people understand. One particular day, I decided to use the bars for a different purpose. I had found a length of poor quality rope and decided to use this rope as a makeshift swing, by tying it onto the monkey bars. I hung it over the bars and tied the ends together forming a loop. I then managed to hang from the bars and swing my legs through the loop and then sat swinging free from the bars. However, because of it's poor quality, the rope didn't have much strength, and it only took about three swings on it before it broke. Naturally, as gravity would have it, I fell down and landed on the concrete base with my head hitting the floor first. Once again I suffered a bad headache and a large lump on the back of my head which also took several days to go down. Luckily there was no cut to my head so I did not have any bleeding, which would have made it look more serious. Again, whether or not I had suffered any concussion was not determined, but I just had to get over it.

My next memory of having more head trauma was during the winter time, although I cannot be specific about the actual date. Whenever we had a fall of snow, it always seemed to be the wet and heavy variety. This was an excellent consistency for us to make an icy slide. We would tamp the snow down with our feet, and rub on it with the soles of our shoes, or boots, which usually had leather soles and heels. When we had finished, we had made ourselves a nice icy slide which could be from 20 to 30 feet long. All the kids would have great fun on these slides, but most times they did not last for more than 2 or 3 days, as the temperature would rise above freezing and the slides would melt away. One evening when one of the slides was still nice and hard, I decided to go out and play on it.

There was no one else around and I was enjoying myself when I tried doing something different. I had seen ice skaters in movies skating on one leg and decided to try it myself. I took a long run toward the slide and began sliding. I then lifted one foot up off the ice behind me and spread my arms out, to help me keep my balance. The next thing I remember was coming 'to', lying on my back at the end of the slide. I had fallen and hit the back of my head on the hard ice and could already feel a lump. I also had a terrible headache. I do not know for how long I had been unconscious. It may have been for only a few seconds but I will never know. Again, there was no cut to my head and therefore no bleeding. When I think about it, ice skaters do not skate on a sloping rink and our slides were made on our street, which was in fact sloping. Maybe this could be why I lost my footing so easily.

I do not remember even telling my mother, or anyone else for that matter, what had happened, as I felt too embarrassed, and again, I could have suffered a concussion and not been treated for it.

It was during one winter time, when we had had the usual fall of wet snow and a few of us were engaged in a snowball fight, that I received a direct hit in my left eye with one of the hard packed snowballs. They used to be packed so firmly that they were more like rounded lumps of ice, and you really knew it if you were hit by one of them. The one that hit my eye just happened to have a stone in the middle of it, which made it that much heavier and hence could inflict more pain on the recipient. I could possibly have had some serious damage to that eye, or even lost the eye altogether, but we seemed to be made of sterner stuff in those days and eventually after a few days of suffering my eye returned to normal, with no apparent permanent damage. My sight was not affected either. It is quite understandable why schools nowadays do not allow children to throw snowballs whilst at school.

There was one incident when another boy and I had had some kind of disagreement and we were going to have a fight over it. We put up our 'dukes' and were sparring with each other, but before either of us had even attempted to hit the other one, this boy's brother sneaked up from behind and 'blindsided' me, swinging a blow at me with his arm fully extended and hitting me full force with his fist on the side of my head. This made my head 'ring' and left me rather dazed, and the original fight never got started. It looked like I must have lost that argument. Incidentally, this particular boy with whom I was going to have the 'scrap' was the same one who had blurted out the question, "What's the name of that road?" when we were attempting to rent the bicycles, mentioned earlier, and I was confident that I could have beaten him in a 'fair' fist fight.

At the time of my next head trauma incident, I think I was about 12 years old. Each week, my mother would give us a treat by taking us to the pictures [movies]. One evening she would take our two sisters and another evening it would be the turn for my brother and myself. As we were walking up our street, heading for the cinema, my brother and I were fooling about, tussling with each other. Of course Charlie was two years older than I, and was consequently bigger also. Hence he would always get the upper hand when we were wrestling with each other. On this particular evening he had managed to get me in a position where I was bent forward with my arms stretched out behind me. He had hold of my wrists and was moving me around like one would push a wheelbarrow, weaving to and fro. My mother was walking ahead of us and did not see what happened next. Although I believe it was not intentional on Charlie's part, he inadvertently 'wheeled' me, head first, straight into the corner edge of a brick wall with reasonable force. My head was 'split open', as the saying goes, and blood was pouring profusely down my face. When my mother turned round to see what all the commotion was about she nearly had a fit. Anyway, despite my protestations she insisted on returning home to, once again, administer medical treatment to me. I of course wanted to carry on to the cinema, and was most disappointed that our treat had to be cancelled. Again there was no thought given to possible concussion. It is a wonder that my head is still in one piece after all the abuse it has received.

Around the same period of time, we used to go to the pictures on a Saturday afternoon to the matinee which was designed for the younger set. There was nearly always a Cowboys and Indians film on, which everyone liked. Anyway, on one Saturday I had gone there sporting a nice new jacket. When I got back home I found that it had a cut all the way down the back. Apparently some hooligan, of which there were many in the queue, had run a razor blade down the back of my coat from top to bottom. We never found out who was responsible. The thought comes to mind that had he pressed a bit harder while vandalising my coat, I could have received a really nasty cut down my back. Luckily that did not happen.

Although we got into all kinds of trouble quite a lot, we very rarely did anything to break the law, but I do remember that when apples were in season we would go into the more 'well to do' areas and 'steal' apples from people's orchards. We used to tuck them into our shirts until we had what looked like a spare tyre all around our waistlines. If any owners saw us we would usually scarper pretty quickly before we got caught, and make our way home, walking, as usual. We enjoyed many apple pies made from our ill gotten gains, because even though our Mothers did not approve of how we got the apples, they could not let them go to waste, and besides we usually only took the windfall apples which would have been left on the ground to rot by the owners. In a way, we were saving the owners a job of cleaning up all the rotten apples. [That, Your Honour, is the case for the defence.]

Gambling was against the Law in those days, and we used to play cards for money, whenever we had any, and the card schools [as they were called] could take place almost anywhere. There was always somebody on look out known as being 'on douse', watching out for any approaching 'Scuffer' [Policeman] who got that nickname from the fact that if anyone was caught by one, 'misbehaving' he would be scuffed over the back of the head, as punishment, so that he would not have to take us to the police station to be charged.

I was once playing Poker with a good pal of mine [Alec Landrum] who lived in the flat above ours, and as money was in short supply we were only playing for halfpennies or pennies. There were only the two of us playing, as this particular day we seemed to be the only ones not at school. There was one 'hand' which has stuck in my head all these years because it was the best Poker hand I have ever had, before or since, [It was 7,8,9,10, J, all of hearts] known as a running flush, or a straight flush, and one of the best hands in Poker. We had both anted up our halfpennies into the kitty and I could not believe my luck in getting such a good hand. It was my turn to bet so I put in a whole penny and waited for Alec to make his bet. I was hoping that at least he would call, by betting another penny so I could collect some reasonable winnings. After perusing his hand he determined that he had nothing of any significance and just folded. So I collected the winnings of my own one and a half pence and Alec's one half penny which meant that with such a fantastic Poker hand I had won the princely sum of one half penny. I would like to think that this must be some sort of record, as probably the smallest amount ever won with a running flush hand in Poker. As I mentioned earlier, this is a Poker hand that I will never forget. About 60 years later, I finally met Alec again when I was visiting England in August 2007, and I mentioned that game to him, but he could not remember it.

It occurs to me, when I look back on those years, that we never went away for a holiday. The nearest thing to a holiday was a day out to the seaside town of New Brighton which was on the other side of the river Mersey over on the Wirral Peninsular, and which had a fine sandy beach. We used to refer to New Brighton as being "over the water". It meant starting out fairly early in the day and it entailed a bus or tram ride down to the Pier Head in Liverpool, followed by a ride on the ferry boat which went across the river. [One may recall the famous song—'Ferry, 'cross the Mersey' sung by Gerry and the Pacemakers]. We, or I should say our Mother, would have to carry a large bag containing such things as cups and various snacks and sandwiches, for us to have something to eat and drink while we were on the beach, as we could not afford to eat out at a café or restaurant, and of course, a towel for each of us.

There was always a stall on the beach from which we could buy a pot tea, and when it was time for tea we would sit on our towels on the sand and munch on our sandwiches. It did not matter what precautions one took, sand particles would always manage to find their way into them and we would end up chewing on what would have now become, 'gritty' sandwiches. If we did not eat them we would just go hungry, so we tucked in anyway.

Usually there were some donkeys on the beach and one could pay to have a ride on them [just a certain distance down the beach and back]. We kids always had a go at that, but I remember one time when my Mother and her friend who lived in the flat below ours and had brought her kids over as well, decided to have a ride on the donkeys. There was a youth who would be in charge of them and would carry a stick to gently smack them to make them move, if they were being stubborn. [The donkeys, that is]. When they had started their ride, my brother Charlie and I were coaxing the youth to hit the donkeys that the two mothers were on, so as to make them break into a trot, as they were only supposed to walk. When he did do so, I can still recall the shrieks that the two ladies gave out, as their donkeys went galloping along the beach. We had a good laugh about that, and were thankful that our Mother did not know that we were the instigators.

When I was ten years old, I was attending school at St. Oswald's Elementary School, in the district of Old Swan, Liverpool. I was in a class of about 25 kids [all boys, as there were no co-ed schools in those days] and we were being primed to take an exam called the 'ELEVEN PLUS'. This was to see if we could qualify to attend a Grammar School which was considered to be a higher education school or College. Most years there were usually about three or four class members who passed the exam and transferred to the College for the following year. In my year there were eight qualifiers, which happened to be the best result ever, and I was one of them. It seems that all the incidents of head trauma that I had suffered, up to that time, had not affected my intellect, but maybe they had knocked some sense into me instead. We were given a choice of two Colleges and I chose St. Francis Xavier's College, [commonly known as S.F.X.]. It was considered quite an achievement to pass the 'scholarship' as the exam was known as. A lot of the students at these Colleges had their tuition paid for by their families, but those who had passed the exam had their tuition fees covered by the local government. I spent the next five years at S.F.X.. and finished school at the age of sixteen. There were a number of reasons for leaving College at that age, but the main one was because we needed some more income into our household. So I left and got myself a job in an office in downtown Liverpool.

This is where I first met Harold Thomas, who was also working in the same office. We were classified as Junior Clerks [a fancy name for Office Boys], and we became good pals and had a friendship which lasted quite a few years, until I had left Littlewoods to emigrate to Canada at age 37. Even though I did visit with him a couple of times while we were vacationing in England, unfortunately, we eventually lost touch with each other.

If I had stayed on in College until I was eighteen I could have gone on to University, but it was not to be. I must say, though, it did feel good to have a job and have some money in my pocket for a change.

There was another noteworthy incident which occurred when I was about 14 years old which could have had serious consequences, for me. Dave Weber, a pal of mine, and I had been to the Pictures [Movies] to the 'first house'. There were two showings, one after the other, and these were known as First or Second 'House'. After the film was over, it was still reasonably early in the evening. All the shops were closed [usually at 5.30. p.m.], but one could still find the Fish and Chip shops open until the patrons had left the cinemas once the Second House was over. [As the years went by and with the advent of the 'Goggle Box' [Television] all the old cinemas were closed down and replaced with Supermarkets and Bingo Halls.] Dave and I decided to get some chips to eat while we were walking home. We could not afford to buy the fish but enjoyed the chips, especially with lots of salt and vinegar on them. When we had finished eating them we crumpled all the wrapping paper, which was mostly newspaper, into a makeshift football and we were dribbling with the 'ball' along the sidewalk and trying to keep possession. At one point when I had the ball, Dave grabbed my arm and pulled me off it. [This would have been classified as a foul in any regular game]. As he pulled me away from the ball, I temporarily lost my balance and staggered across the sidewalk crashing backwards into a big plate glass window of one of the shops [which, luckily, was closed.] The window shattered and I landed on my backside on the window ledge. As I 'plonked' down, a huge pointed shard of the glass fell from the top of the window and dropped down right next to me, missing me by just a few inches, and smashed into pieces on the sidewalk. If I had been about a foot or so further to my right this large pointed shard of glass would have hit me point first right in my back and one can only speculate as to what the outcome might have been. [That plate glass was pretty heavy]. As it turned out I did not incur any cuts or bruises whatsoever, and I considered myself extremely lucky to have come out of this totally unscathed.

There was quite a lot of noise as the glass smashed on the sidewalk and Dave and I looked up and down the street quickly, to see if anyone had heard all the commotion. As there were very few people about because all the regular shops were closed, nobody seemed to have noticed anything, so Dave and I took to our heels and fled the scene. We ran down one of the adjacent streets, cut through a back entry, and returned to the main road up the next street where we just started walking normally, away from the scene, as if nothing had happened. [A crafty move]. Of course we never did own up about it, and we were never suspected of being involved. I imagine that the store owner would have been compensated under the vandalism clause in his insurance policy.

Although this incident could have had a potentially fatal outcome for me, I am not including it in my list of narrow escapes from death. It was just another dangerous situation, from which I luckily escaped unharmed.

It was while I was still 14 years old when I "borrowed" my Dad's bike to go riding with my pals. This was what my Dad used to ride to work and back, but as it was Sunday he was having a 'lie in'. So I took the bike thinking we would be riding to the park a couple of miles away. Instead we went on an adventure a bit further afield, that took us through the Mersey Tunnel which went under the River Mersey, and came out on the Wirral Peninsular at Birkenhead. The river Mersey is about 1 mile wide, but because of the tunnel having the long sloping entrance and exit, the actual distance one had to travel from one end to the other was nearer to 2 miles.

The biggest problem with this venture was that bikes were not allowed to be ridden through the tunnel as it was considered rather dangerous. The angle of the gradient was very steep at both entrance and exit and as we proceeded down into the tunnel our bikes picked up speed and we seemed to <u>hurtle</u> down to the bottom where the tunnel flattened out and carried on underneath the river. If we had lost control of the steering we could have been badly injured. I remember a taxi passing me and just missing the handlebars of my bike by about 6 inches. It does not bear thinking about what would have happened if the taxi had clipped the handlebars. Incidentally, passing was not allowed in the tunnel, but then again our bikes were not allowed in there either. The experience was so scary that when it was time to go back home we decided to take the Ferry Boat from Birkenhead to Liverpool, where, upon arriving home, I faced the wrath of my Dad for taking his bike without permission. After all, the bike was his mode of transport to and from work, and it could have ended up as a clump of mangled metal, apart from the possibility that I could have been severely injured or even killed in an accident, and ended up as a clump of mangled bones. Once again I came through another potentially dangerous situation unscathed, but, in my opinion, not a serious enough incident to be included in my lucky escapes from death.

5

During my younger years I cannot remember ever having a tooth brush, so it should not be surprising that, with our diet over the years, which always seemed to include lots of sugar and sweets and toffees, our teeth eventually suffered. The only time I can remember going to the Dentist was when we were taken by the school, when I was about six years old, and as far as I know, I hadn't seen one since. Well, here I was, now sixteen and having <u>serious</u> trouble with my teeth and was forced to pluck up the courage to go and see a Dentist. When my teeth were examined, the Dentist informed me that they were in a pitiful condition and that all of my back teeth, both top and bottom, were in various stages of <u>bad</u> decay, so much so that he recommended that I should have them all extracted. An appointment was made and I eventually turned up on the fateful day that the surgery was to be performed. It was considered to be fairly major surgery because I was having twelve back teeth out in one session.

In those days for most serious dental work, gas was always used, and as it was preferable to complete the work in one visit, a lot of gas was used in order that I would remain anaesthetized long enough for the work to be finished. These days they have what is called 'Sedation Dentistry', but I am sure it is not quite the same thing.

After I was put 'under' I had no idea how long I was out for, but this is what I recall for the period I was out. It felt like I was dreaming and I was floating along over an undulating landscape which was covered with lush green grass and lots of colourful flowers and I felt very calm and happy. This confirms for me that one can dream in colour. This floating went on for what seemed only a short while, then all of a sudden I seemed to be in the Dentist's office, but I was floating up in the corner of the ceiling. A Dentist's chair was in the centre of the room and there were two people in white coats attending a patient in the chair. I couldn't see who it was but I had a strong sensation that it was me in that chair. I could not hear anything either. Even though I was in what was a small room for the surgery, the two attendants seemed to be quite a distance away and appeared to be a lot smaller as a result.

After what was seemingly another short period of time, every thing went completely black and I have no conception as to how long this lasted. Suddenly I could see a tiny white dot of light that seemed to be a long distance away and I felt like I was rushing towards it. When I finally reached the dot of light it suddenly became a large circle of light and it felt like I was coming out of a tunnel. As I came out into the light, my eyes opened and I was still in the Dentist's chair with somebody slapping my face as if they were trying to bring me round. I can only assume that I had undergone what is known as an 'out of body' experience, and that I had been having difficulty getting back into my body, hence the slapping of my face to bring me round, by one of the white coated attendants. I had read of cases during that era where dental patients, who were given heavy doses of gas for lengthy surgery, did not recover from it, and I am surmising that I very nearly became another statistic.

I am not sure whether or not my 'out of body' experience would be considered as a brush with death, but the way events happened while I was 'out,' and the history of fatalities in such situations, it definitely seemed like a near miss to me, so I do count it as my <u>fifth</u> lucky escape from death.

It was while I was still sixteen that there was a period in my life when my artistic nature came to the fore and lasted for about two years, until I was conscripted into the Armed Forces for my mandatory two years service. It took the form of Ballroom Dancing. My friend Harold Thomas and myself were no different from any other teenage boys. We liked to try to pick up girls and we thought that one good way to meet girls was on the River Cruise ferry boat, the Royal Iris. The boat used to cruise up the river Mersey to the bar and back, and on board they held a dance for the duration of the cruise. We thought that this would be good 'hunting' grounds for the purpose. So, one Saturday evening, we went on one of the cruises and ventured into the dance hall to try our hands, as it were [or should that be feet]. However, neither of us had any idea of how to dance, and when we saw all the couples dancing and doing all their fancy steps, we could only stand and gape in awe. Hence, neither of us could pluck up the courage to ask any of the girls to dance, for fear of showing ourselves up. So the bright idea turned out to be a failure. We both, then and there, resolved to learn to dance and to that end we both joined a dancing school to learn ballroom dancing. It took some courage for us to do that, but as there were two of us it made it a little easier. I remember the name of the school was The Skelland School of Dancing which was situated in Ullet Road in Liverpool and was about half way between where we each lived. We attended diligently for several months and after learning some basic steps to a number of dances, we thought we would try the River Cruise once more. So, when we did go on the Cruise, we once again ventured into the dance hall. We stood for a few minutes and watched the dancers, who, in our now 'knowledgeable' opinion were doing a 'load of rubbish' as far as dance steps go. Everyone who got onto the dance floor just seemed to shuffle about and tried to move in time with the music. Hardly anybody was dancing properly according to how our dance lessons had taught us.

So once again we felt a bit out of our depth. I can't recall whether we actually did dance on that cruise or not, and I am pretty sure that we didn't pick up any of the girls either.

I can remember an amusing anecdote that was posted on the wall above the urinals in the men's room on the Royal Iris ferry boat. It read "We aim to please.... You aim <u>too</u>, please".

The one thing that we both agreed on was that we both enjoyed the dancing at the dance studio, so we started to go there on a regular basis and got to like it so much that we used to go six evenings a week. If that wasn't enough we used to attend what was known as a 'Tea Dance' at a local dance hall [called The Rialto] on each Saturday afternoon. When the band took a break there would be complimentary tea and biscuits [cookies] for the patrons. Hence the name 'Tea Dance'. We found that on the Saturday afternoons there were not very many people at the dance hall which was quite convenient for us, as there was lots of room on the dance floor for us to practice our dances and variations that we had been taught throughout the week. We were both very keen students and we became quite proficient and consequently we got a lot of enjoyment from it.

Although we danced with lots of girls at the local dance hall we never seemed to 'pick up' any of them and anyway all our evenings were taken up by going to the dance studio. I used to like it so much that once in a while I also gave a helping hand in the teaching of new students. Both Harold and myself had reached Silver Medal standard by the time we were whisked off to defend Queen and Country. Being conscripted into the Armed Forces put an end to that phase of my life, but the memory of that time and the enjoyment I got from it are still fondly remembered. Of course the fact that we had learned to dance gave us more confidence in later years whenever we attended any functions where there was dancing included. One never forgets how to do most things that we are taught; it's like riding a bike, as the saying goes. Of course, as time passes, the type or style of dancing changes and if one doesn't keep apprised of the constant changing, one tends to get left behind and seemingly out of one's depth yet again.

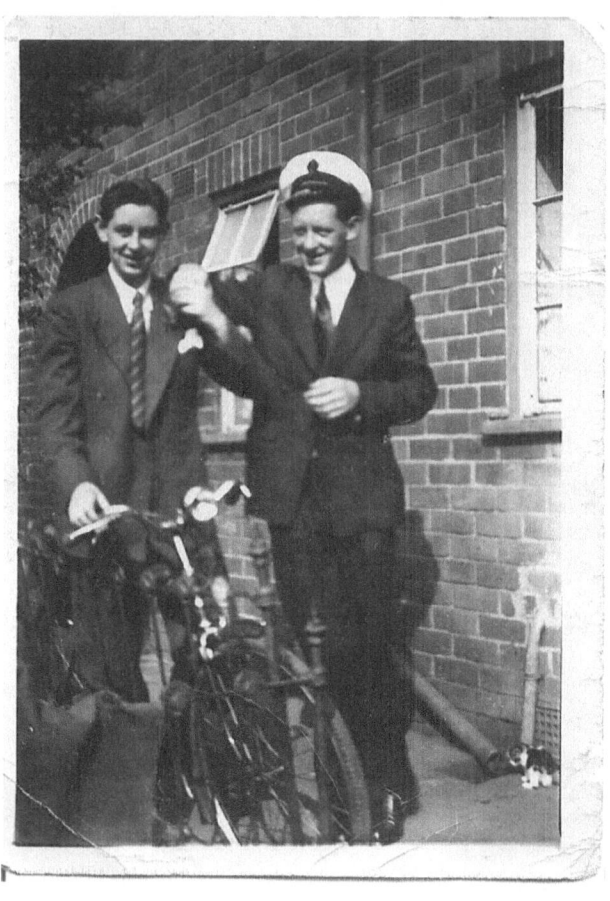

William Carroll [astride bike] with my brother Charlie, who was in his Royal Navy Uniform. Charlie was nineteen years old and I was seventeen, some months prior to my being called up to do my two years compulsory National Service.

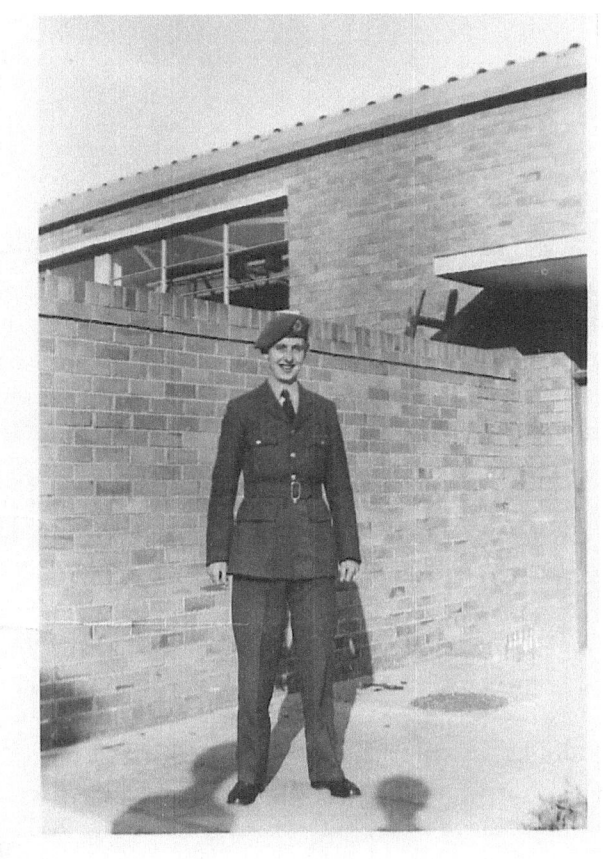

A photo of William Carroll [The author] taken in 1953, at age eighteen, in R.A.F. uniform, while on leave in Liverpool, England. [Note the shiny shoes].

6

As history shows, World War 2 ended in 1945, but because Britain was so unprepared for war in 1939 it was decided to carry on conscripting young men into the armed forces, so that we should be more prepared in the future. This continued for several years after the War's end and when I reached 18 years of age, it was my turn to be conscripted. The year was 1953 and I think conscription ended in 1955.

Everyone who was 'called up' had to undergo a medical exam, and all those who passed went on to the next stage which was to be inoculated, although we were not told what it was for. One friend of mine was in line awaiting his turn for the needle. When he got near to the front of the line he saw the doctor stick the needle into someone's arm and it made him feel ill, so much so that he actually fainted. This was reason enough for him to be given a low medical grading and he was rejected as Forces material. There was another lad that I knew who was rejected because he had flat feet. All the selection process was taking place in a large building in down town Liverpool, and presumably all other big cities would have had similar processing centres.

There were three branches of the armed forces that we had the choice of joining; namely, the Army, Navy, or Air Force. Those who chose the Army had no problem and were signed up right away, but if one chose either of the other two branches he would be marshalled into a classroom where, along with others who had chosen the same branch, he would have to sit at a desk and complete an intelligence test. If anyone didn't reach a certain standard, he would be told that he would have to go into the Army. This is not to infer that all the recruits going into the Army were of lower intellect. There were plenty of people who were a bit leery about flying or sailing in boats who chose the Army in the first place. I had elected to join the Air Force and managed to pass their test. [Dare I say—with 'flying' colours?]

Soon after [just a few weeks], we were actually 'called up' and ordered to report to certain camps at which we would be kitted out and further assessed to see which training camp we would be assigned to. After arriving at this first camp, at Padgate, I remember that I had only one shilling and six pence in my pocket. The next morning we were all marched off to the barber shop where we all had our hair cut, even though I had had mine cut just two days earlier. The hair cut cost me one shilling which left me with only six pence in my pocket. As I had started smoking cigarettes and did not have enough money to buy any, I 'borrowed' tuppence [two pence] from a fellow recruit in my hut and bought 5 'woodies' [Woodbine cigarettes]. One could buy a packet of 5 in those days, which cost eight pence. [Just over 3 new pence.]

Most of the other fellows had arrived at the camp with adequate supplies of cash and here was I, now broke and waiting for pay-day which was 5 or 6 days away. When I think back to this hair cut 'lark' I feel it must have been some sort of scam, as I am not quite sure that it was mandatory and that the corporal who took us there must have had some 'arrangement' with the barber shop. Of course we all had to 'obey orders' and get our hair cut, whether we needed it or not. [It was easy money for the Barber Shop.]

When we were all kitted out, we were posted to our training camps according to various criteria. [Mainly education level and experience]. I was sent to a camp at a place called Hednesford where the recruits were classified as P.O.M's [potential officer material]. However, one could only become an officer if he was prepared to apply for 'air crew', but as I had a fear of flying, and did not apply for 'air crew' I ended up as a common 'airman' and a member of 'ground crew'. Why did I apply for the Air Force? [One might ask].

During the six weeks at Hednesford we were put through what is known as 'square bashing', which consisted of: Marching and drill routines, [on the barrack square] assault courses, firearms and fitness training, and various lectures. I had discovered that there was a friend of mine [Harold Thomas] at the same camp, and he was already two weeks into his training. I used to go and visit him in the evenings and he would show me various drills that we would be encountering. Hence, I was always ahead of the game and consequently good at our drill sessions.

As often happens, in most groups of people there are always one or two 'odd ball' characters, and my group was no exception. Out of the 20 or so in my billet there were two of these. The first one could never seem to get the hang of marching. Each time we were on parade there was always some marching to be done, and this fellow would always swing his right arm forward at the same time as his right foot was stepping forward. Similarly, he would do the same with his left arm and left foot. No matter how many times he was shown how to march properly he still could never get it right. I don't remember if he finally got it or not.

The second guy had the habit of always calling the Corporal instructor 'Sergeant' and the Corporal was getting a bit annoyed with him. So, one morning, during our usual drill instruction, the Corporal called him out front and their conversation went like this:-
Corporal ... "Airman, how many stripes does a <u>Sergeant</u> have on his sleeve?"
Airman.... "Three, Sergeant"
Corporal ... "And how many stripes do <u>I</u> have on <u>my</u> sleeve?"
Airman ... "Two, Sergeant."

I think the Corporal just gave up on him, and I never noticed whether or not the Airman finally understood. He probably had a bad case of nerves which caused him to be confused.

About a week into our training we all had to have some injections. I can't remember what they were for, but they were given in two stages. Apparently, the first one was a weaker version of the second one, to get us accustomed to whatever it was, before we received the stronger dose. We just knew them as the 25's and 75's. After the first injection, everyone, except myself, was complaining of soreness and pain around the injection site. Some had a bad rash while others had swelling of the area but all were suffering to some extent. There were a few who could not even bear their shirt sleeves to rub on the site, as it was so sensitive. I could not understand what all the fuss and bother was about, as my arm was completely normal and I was slapping it and saying, "there's nothing wrong with my arm"

However, the next morning, as with every morning at this camp, we had to go out on parade and be marched to the mess hall for breakfast. We were lined up as usual with our pint sized earthenware mugs [for tea] and irons [stainless steel knife, fork, and spoon] clasped in our hands behind our backs, standing in the 'at ease' position. Most of the group were still moaning and groaning about their arms, while mine still felt normal. The next thing I remember, I came to, lying on my back with a ring of faces looking down at me. I had apparently just collapsed and had fallen straight back, still in the 'at ease' position. My mug was smashed under my back. The explanation as to what had happened was that instead of the effects of the injection manifesting themselves by coming out on my arm, as with the rest of the group, in my case the effects had gone inwards and had caused me to 'black out' [faint]. Luckily, with my mug being smashed under my back, no sharp pieces of it had managed to pierce my back, nor had I fallen awkwardly onto my knife. Also, it was possible that I could have suffered a concussion, as I did bang my head on the ground as I fell and I remember having quite a bad headache as a result of it. I could have been severely injured had any of these things happened. However, I was helped back into the barrack room, where I lay on my bed to recuperate, and I didn't seem to have any ill effects in the days following. Of course the most important thing on my mind at the time was that I had missed breakfast. Because of all the physical activity we were put through, it seemed that we were always hungry and, even after our evening meal, we would always end up a couple of hours later in the 'NAAFI' buying some more food to keep us going until breakfast the next morning.

The stronger injection, which was administered a few days later, seemed to have no ill effects on me at all. Apparently, the earlier, weaker, injection must have done its job, despite the unfortunate effect that it had had on me.

This was just another incident, in my life, although somewhat quite dangerous, that I am not including in my list of lucky escapes from death.

After we had finished our six weeks of 'square bashing' and we had all qualified, we were given our postings to various camps where we were to do our 'trade' training. Some of us were sent to Middle Wallop in Wiltshire, England where we trained as 'fighter plotters'. After completing the course satisfactorily, I was posted to a camp in the North East of England where I spent the best part of my two years service. This camp, called Seaton Snook, had a large underground Radar Station, complete with an operations room, where I did most of my work.

Looking back, my earliest recollection of suffering from Hay Fever was when I was just seven years old, playing in the tall grass in the park in Liverpool. One nice Spring day, while still posted at Seaton Snook, a few of us had walked a couple of miles into the seaside town of Seaton Carew, while we were off duty, and it was on the way back that we noticed that the grass was being cut all over the camp. As we got closer, I suddenly had a very severe bout of Hay Fever. It was the worst attack that I had ever experienced and I began to have great difficulty in breathing, just like an asthmatic attack. It was so bad that I couldn't even walk over a small hump backed bridge. The next morning I reported 'sick' and had an appointment with the camp's Medical Officer. After hearing of my difficulty in breathing, he gave me a Doctors Note which excused me from attending parades or from marching. Of course, because we were put through our paces quite strenuously the whole time we were at this camp, it was a relief for me to have this Doctors Note, so that I could legitimately avoid some of the stressful activities for a while, at least until the hay fever season was over.

The camp had a 'Tuck Shop' which provided such things as, tea, biscuits [cookies], chocolate bars etc. and a place to relax when we were off duty, just like a Coffee Bar, [although it didn't provide any coffee]. Naturally, one had to pay for all these items and I remember that even though the price of the cups of tea was quite low, it afforded the highest profit of all the items. I reckoned that the mark-up was as high as 300% to 400%, or maybe even more.

It was during my second year at the camp and I was working my shift at the Tuck Shop, as we all had to do, and I was due to go on leave as soon as I was finished. Everything went quite smoothly and I duly handed over the responsibilities of the job to the airman who was taking over from me, and promptly left for home. A couple of days into my leave I received a letter requesting my return to camp, to attend an inquiry into a shortage of funds from the Tuck Shop. There was also a railway warrant included with the letter. When I got back to the camp and was questioned about the missing money, all I could do was state that when I had handed things over to the next shift worker, everything had tallied and it was accepted that I had followed procedure correctly. Therefore, I was no longer under suspicion regarding the shortage and was allowed to return home to finish my leave. I was also allowed an extra day to be added to my leave to compensate for the disruption. It must have looked very suspicious on my part, considering the timing of my departure was right after finishing my shift at the Tuck Shop. I understand that the airman who took over from me was eventually found to be the culprit, but I never heard if he had been charged for the offence or what punishment, if any, was meted out to him.

In all of the armed forces there is a system whereby recruits are punished for minor misdemeanors [such as dirty buttons, bedspace not spotless, turning up late for parade etc.] by being confined to camp. Each morning of the period of confinement they have to report to the guard room carrying full 'field kit' which weighs about 100 lbs. Each day, for three or four hours, the 'offenders' would be put through some harsh and physically draining routines. Usually the punishment period would be for only a few days and in the R.A.F. [during my time] it was known as doing 'JANKERS'. Other branches of the forces each have their own nickname for it.

Virtually all recruits get charged with some minor offence or other during their term of service and have to do a few days of 'JANKERS'. It seemed like the N.C.O.'s went out of their way to find something to charge us with. Luckily, or cunningly, I managed to avoid any such punishment during my two years and consequently I can make an unusually rare <u>boast</u> about it.

After I was demobbed from the Air Force I returned to Liverpool and resumed my old job with The Road Haulage Executive known as the B.R.S. [The British Road Services] and life continued on in its usual hum-drum way. Eventually I acquired a position with Littlewoods in the Head Office of their Retail business, [about a hundred Department Stores, and several Catalogue Companies.] It was a job as part of one of several teams charged with keeping adequate stocks of goods balanced as to colours and sizes in some or all of the various outlets, working closely with various manufacturers. It was a job which I thoroughly enjoyed and I was to spend about fourteen years at this company, obtaining several promotions on the way, before my life would take a dramatic turn. But more about that later.

Incidentally, the friend who was at the square bashing camp, two weeks ahead of me, Harold Thomas, was also working for Littlewoods, but as mentioned earlier, after I left the firm we lost touch with each other. He eventually became an Executive Director of the company.

A few years after resuming civilian life we moved house, that is to say, we moved from our flat to a two storey house about two miles further out from town. It was a couple of years later that I first met Lilian [my wife to be] who happened to live in the same neighbourhood. The circumstances of our first encounter were a little unusual and not without a bit of humour. I was off work 'sick' one day and had an appointment with my Doctor at a time which meant I found myself at the bus stop at the same time as Lil, who was on her way to work. We did not know each other except by sight, [but we did admire each other from afar] and on a whim, I decided to get on the same bus as her and 'chat her up' [which took a lot of courage on my part]. The bus she needed took a different route to town but I got on it anyway. The bus was pretty crowded as it was still rush hour, and there were very few seats available. Lil managed to find one and sat down and I stood next to her and started talking to her. The contents of our conversation elude me now, but it ended up with my making a date with her for that evening. As I needed to get off the bus after a few stops I left saying "I'll see you tonight" and "By the way, what's your name?" Lil said later that she had felt terribly embarrassed because all the passengers in the near vicinity were hanging on our every word. Thus we began going out together.

I found out shortly after, that Lilian had also passed the 'scholarship' and had attended an all girls Grammar School, called Broughton Hall College for Young Ladies. So, we were both considered to be worthy of a higher education and I attribute this to the fact that our three kids all turned out to be very bright and they did us both proud when they all went on to complete a university education, with excellent results.

A few months after we had started courting, I was walking Lilian home to her house one evening after she had been to visit our house for tea, [commonly known as supper in North America] when she noticed something across the road and said "Look at that". As she said it I turned towards her to see where she was looking. At that precise moment she happened to point towards the object, and her finger poked me in my eye, causing me considerable pain. As I was holding my eye and wincing from the pain, Lil broke down in a fit of laughter and thought the incident was hilarious. I obviously didn't <u>see</u> the humour in it [literally] and 'took the huff', because she did not appreciate the distress I was in. Nor was there any apology for inflicting this pain on me. I turned and ungallantly walked away from her and returned to my house, leaving her to walk home by herself. She lived only a few blocks away. Because of that juvenile tantrum of mine we very nearly broke up and I never did find out what it was that she had noticed. A couple of days later Lil came round to our house to pick something up, which she had left there. When she had gone, I ran after her to try to patch things up. Luckily, we got back together again, and within a couple of years we were married [October 1963]. I often reflect on that 'finger in the eye' incident and thank my lucky stars that I had the courage to try and patch things up between us. If I hadn't done that we would not have got to enjoy our lovely honeymoon on the isle of Majorca nor been blessed with our three great kids. [Andrew, Michael, and Alison.]

Whenever this 'finger' story is related, at family get togethers, it always gives rise to a few laughs. [By the females, of course].

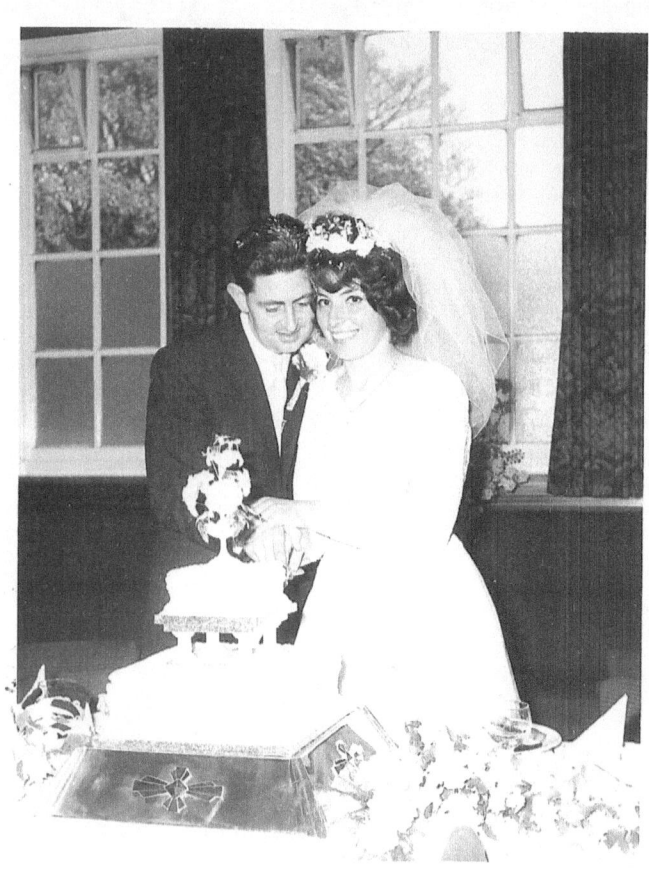

A picture of Lilian and myself at our wedding reception Oct. 1963 in Liverpool, England.

[Happier times]

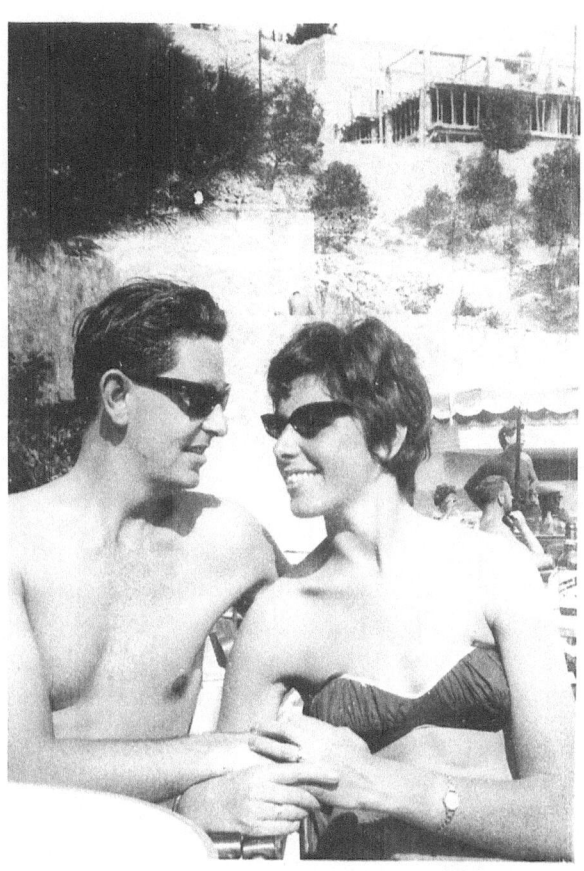

William and Lilian enjoying the nice weather while on their honeymoon on the isle of Majorca, just off the east coast of Spain, in the Balearic Islands, Oct. 1963.

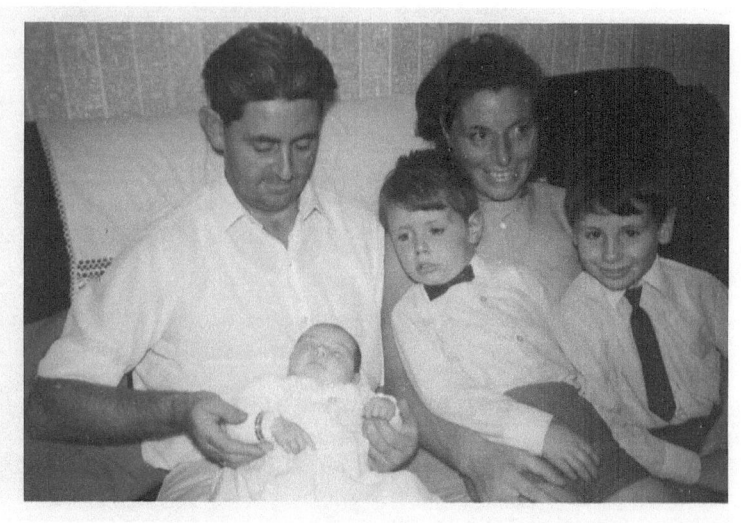

Lilian and William, in their home in Prescot, England, with their young family [from Right to Left] Andrew, Michael and Alison in August 1970, just after Alison's christening. Two years after this picture was taken they had all emigrated to Calgary, Canada.

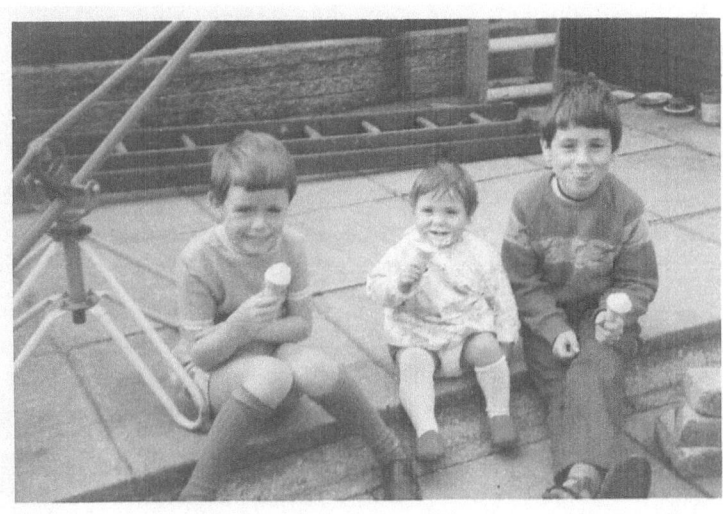

From left to right:-Michael, Alison and Andrew, enjoying icecream cornets in our back garden in Prescot in Sept. 1971. Ten months after this picture was taken we were all on our way to Calgary, Canada to start our new lives, [July 1972]

All three of our kids were born while we were living in the house which we had bought in Prescot just outside of Liverpool, and we stayed in that house for just over eight years, when we eventually emigrated to Canada. There are a few interesting things which happened during our stay in Prescot that I would like to relate, some of which might well have been quite serious while others may have had a little humour to them, depending on which side of the incident you were on. Andrew, our first baby, was born in 1964, Michael our second, in 1966. Six months after Michael's birth something very serious happened to Lil. She had started to bleed badly, so much so, that I had run down to the phone box at the end of our street to call for an ambulance to take her to the emergency at Whiston Hospital. (Many people did not have phones in their houses then, as they do now). At one stage, because of the enormous amount of blood loss, the doctor could not find any blood pressure reading, at all, and she had to be given lots of blood transfusions. Things were so bad that we nearly lost her, but fortunately Lil eventually recovered thanks to the diligence of the emergency medical team. If this problem had not occurred, we would have had another baby boy, but with Lil's body obviously not being ready for another one, the baby was unfortunately lost. Alison was born three and a half years later, in 1970.

All in all, we lived a pretty normal family life and we used to take two holidays each year, always within the U.K. One would usually be for two weeks in the summer time, and the other for just one week in late Autumn.

I must recount three occasions when I unintentionally 'ill-treated' our three kids, at different times of course. All of them were [or could have been] serious at the time, but we can laugh about them now.

When Andrew was just a few weeks old, Lil had put him in his pram outside the front door to get some fresh air. I was 'on duty' looking after him, and was sitting on the front step, pushing the pram to and fro on the path which ran along the front of the house and continued down the side of the house. Lil called for me to come in for something, so I left the pram and went in. After a couple of minutes we heard Andrew crying faintly, and I was about to go and see to him. Lil said, "Leave him, hard as it may be, we can't go running to him every time he cries". So we left him for a few more minutes, and I went back out to carry on my 'duties'. The pram was not outside the front door where I had left it. What had happened was that when I had left it to go inside I had failed to put the brake on and there was a breeze blowing across the front of the house, which was strong enough to move the pram along the path. It had rolled along to the end of the house where the path made a right angled turn to go down the side of the house, and had tipped off the edge. Andrew had slid forward and had been thrown out of the pram and was lying face down in the grass. Had he been thrown about six inches further, his face would have landed on the wire fencing [just lengths of wire between the posts] and he could have been seriously injured. Also, he might have been smothered with his face flat on the grass. Luckily, he was all right, as he was tightly bundled up, and after that incident we tended to go to him each time he cried, especially as he was usually quite docile and didn't cry much at all. Within the next year I had paved-in the driveway from the sidewalk up to and right along the side of the house, so that this sort of accident couldn't happen again.

It was about four years later, when Michael was two years old, that it was his turn for a bit of "ill-treatment" [inadvertently, of course]. We were on holiday somewhere in Wales, and we were all out walking one day. Michael was ahead of me and, as I had done many times before, I came up behind him and went to pick him up by holding him under his elbows. Instead of keeping his arms tucked in to his sides, which is the best way to lift someone up, he let his arms lift up behind him making it impossible for me to lift him properly. I had already raised his feet off the ground and instead of lifting him up I unavoidably threw him forward. We just happened to be walking along a gravel pathway at the time, and poor Michael landed on his face in the gravel. He sustained multiple scrapes down one side of his face. Of course I felt terrible and if anyone had seen it happen, it would have looked like it had been done deliberately. We took him into a local Chemist shop [Pharmacy] where they treated his wounds and after wiping away all the blood, his injuries didn't look as severe as they did at first. Fortunately, he healed fairly quickly and there was no permanent scarring.

Approximately two more years down the road Alison had her turn of apparent "ill-treatment". She was only a few weeks old and was asleep in her cot upstairs at home in Prescot. Lil asked me to bring her downstairs, probably to be fed, so I went up as requested to get her. When I reached into the cot to pick her up, I got hold of her arms just above the elbows and attempted to 'lever' her up by them. It was then that one of her shoulder joints dislocated. I can't remember exactly what happened after that. There was a bit of a panic and Lil came to the rescue and saved the day, and Alison's shoulder joint went back into place. We took her to the hospital where they put her arm in a sling, but there was no sign of any ill effects, immediately following, or in the years to follow. Of course I was called a few 'choice' names by Lil for my 'stupidity'.

Every family must go through some rough patches where accidents like these happen and eventually it became my turn to have some mishaps, a couple of which I remember quite well. At the time of the first mishap, Andrew was 5 and Michael was 3, and we were playing football [soccer] on our front lawn. There was a low brick wall, about 2 feet high, which bordered the front edge of the lawn adjacent to the sidewalk, and which had very rough edges. Of course I was running rings around them showing off my dribbling skills. At one point the ball was kicked over the wall into the street. I naturally just jumped over the wall to retrieve it. I threw the ball back onto the lawn and took a run at the wall to jump back over it. However, I managed to misjudge the wall's height by about one inch and caught the toe of my leading foot on the top edge of it. As Physics would have it, my weight was already committed and I carried on over the wall, but because of my toe's being caught, I fell forward over the wall with my legs trailing behind. One of my legs happened to scrape down the rough edge and I received a bad gash down my shin, which bled profusely and caused me considerable pain. Both boys said, "Are you alright Dad?". I just rubbed Michael's head as I was passing him and hobbled quickly indoors, where I let out the loud yell that I had been holding in. Lil thought it was all quite humourous but she managed to stifle her amusement while she tended my wound. She told me later that I had gone all pale, probably from the shock. Unfortunately that mishap ended my play session with our two boys.

Some weeks later I was watching Andrew and Michael playing in the back garden, when I set the wheels in motion for my next mishap to take place. I had recently built a retaining wall along the front edge of the back lawn and filled in behind it to level the lawn, which was originally sloping down towards the house. They had placed two of the left over house bricks on the lawn, side by side, and were running and jumping over them. However, Michael, being only 3, was not doing it 'right'. He was running up to the bricks and stopping. Then he would take a big step over them, instead of jumping over them. I went outside to show him how he should do it and then I suggested another way to use the bricks. I said to them "Try doing it this way". I placed the bricks one on top of the other and stood with my feet together just in front of them. The object was to jump over the bricks with both feet together. As I took a leap across them, I had not realised that a washing line was stretching across the lawn in line with the bricks, high enough for the boys to not be hampered by it, but not so for me. As I jumped, the line caught me under my chin. Once again my body was committed to moving forward and being restrained at the chin, I pivoted around that point when Gravity took over and I fell down with my back landing on the bricks. As luck would have it I didn't sustain any noticeable injury, even though I could have broken my back. I think my pride suffered more damage than my body. Although they didn't know it, our two boys had just seen another Physics experiment being performed. The only comment that I got from them was Andrew saying "Couldn't we just do it our way, Dad?" When will parents ever learn to leave kids to make their <u>own</u> fun?

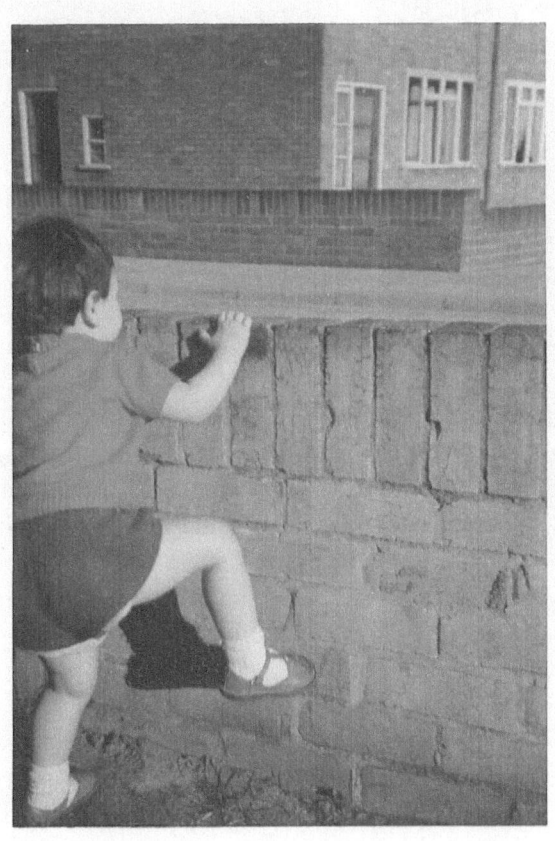

This picture shows Andrew trying to climb the low wall which was bordering our front lawn. It was the wall that I [William] was destined to fall over and gash my shin on, when I was retrieving the ball from the street.

7

At this particular point, I would like to mention how my family and I decided to emigrate to Canada.

Some years earlier, my older sister Betty, at age 21, had married her husband Charl, and not too long afterwards, they had a baby daughter, Janice. A couple of years later they decided to emigrate to Canada [to Calgary, Alberta] where there was lots of opportunity for a better life. Every few years they would revisit England for a few weeks vacation, and while they were 'back home' Betty would always be expounding the virtues of life in Canada and trying to encourage us to make the break, and move over there ourselves.

We were quite happy with our life in England, and had resisted Betty's attempts to convince us, so far. We were getting along just fine in our home in Prescot. My job at Littlewoods was very demanding, but was also very rewarding and it paid quite well. I had had advancements over the years and on my next promotion I would be entitled to a company car and, best of all, a parking space under our building, [an envied prize in downtown Liverpool]. However, there had been a change in management and someone had been brought in over our heads to take charge of the department I was in. There was an uneasy atmosphere about the place after he took over and I just couldn't seem to get on with him. At that time the Company had adopted the more psychological approach to personnel management, just like businesses were doing in the U.S.A., and this presented me with a dilemma. I could not work with this new manager and I instinctively knew that he would not recommend me for that desired next promotion. Also, because of the psychological approach that the Personnel Department was taking, it would be futile to request a transfer to another department as that would be tantamount to admitting that I could not resolve the problem of the clash of personalities between myself and the newly inducted manager. In their eyes this meant that I would not be 'suitable management material'. Result-stalemate!

Shortly after, Betty and Charl were over again visiting 'back home' and she was again trying to encourage us to move over to Canada. Lil and I had a talk later on, when we were on our own, and discussed my situation at work. I just couldn't go on working with the new manager indefinitely, waiting for him to move on, and I new that I couldn't expect any further advancement while he was my manager, so we decided that we should give it a try in Canada. It was quite a big step for us to take, especially with our having three children [ages, 7, 5, & 1], and I really hated to leave my job. It is unfortunate that despite liking a job, one also has to get on with the other people with whom one has to work, particularly the Manager, in order to enjoy it and be successful at it.

To cut a long story short, we were processed for eligibility as immigrants for Canada, and acquired sufficient points to be accepted. We all had to undergo full medical examinations, at our own expense, and we were all given a clean bill of health. I recall one amusing moment when I was having my eyes tested. The nurse who was checking them asked me to read the bottom line on the chart. It made me squint a bit, but I eventually got it and read out "Made in England". I was of course reading the place where the chart had been produced and printed, which information was written on the bottom of the chart below [and smaller than] the lines of test letters. Needless to say my eyes were declared to be satisfactory.

We had previously agreed with Betty, that we could stay with them when we came over, until I could get a job and we could purchase our own house. I expected that we could give it a couple of weeks for us to settle in and familiarise ourselves with our surroundings, and then I would get myself a job, and in no time we would be in our own house. It took a bit longer than we thought it would, and it was actually about six months before things worked out, but things sorted themselves out eventually and we settled in quite well, even though the pangs of 'homesickness' bothered us for some time.

Lilian had affirmed, and I had agreed, that we would give it at least two years to see how our move worked out, because there had been lots of instances in the past when immigrants were unable to settle down quickly enough, and ended up going back to England, only to realise as soon as they arrived back there, that they had made a mistake and promptly made arrangements to return to Canada. This scenario was well known and was given the nickname of 'The thousand dollar cure'. Luckily we did not fall into that particular trap, and we <u>made</u> things work out. We decided that in our third year we would take a holiday back 'home', and that is what we did. We thoroughly enjoyed it, but were still pleased to be returning to our new home in Calgary, when the holiday was over.

It was within the second year after we had arrived in Canada that the following incident happened in our back yard that could have had serious consequences for our family, if it weren't for the intervention of Andrew, our then 9 year old son. We had been in our own house for just over a year.

We had purchased a rather old car, as we really needed a vehicle to get around, having 3 small kids and all. It used to run okay generally, but one day there was an electrical problem under the hood and I decided to try to correct it myself. I drove the car along the back lane to the back of the house where there was enough room to drive it onto our back yard area and I stopped it at about 8 or 9 feet from the back steps, which were comprised of a concrete block which was about 2ft 6ins high. I parked the car and left the engine running. Andrew had come with me to see if he could be of some help and I left him sitting in the front seat.

I raised the hood and while the car was idling I was attempting to adjust something [I can't remember the name of the part]. I asked Andrew to move over to the driver's seat and put his foot on the accelerator pedal to get the engine to run faster while I did the adjustment. As he did so, the car suddenly slipped its gears and went into 'Drive' mode. As this happened the car surged forward towards me and I was between it and the concrete steps. I must have jumped back before the car could hit me, I just don't remember. Andrew, although he was only 9 years old, had the presence of mind to quickly push the gear lever [which was on the steering column] into the 'Park' position, as he had seen me do whenever we had stopped the car. The car ground to a halt and this all happened in what seemed like a split second.

It was only then that I realised my position. The car had come to a stop at approximately 2ft 6ins from the concrete steps and I was still between it and the steps. If Andrew had not acted as quickly as he did, the car would have hit the concrete block and I would have had my legs crushed in the process, at just about knee height which was the height of the front bumper on the car, [which weighed about two tons.]

This was one occasion when a young child had wanted to help his dad, and in doing so, he most probably saved his dad from losing his legs. If my legs had been lost, what a drastic and devastating change it would have made in our lives. It doesn't bear thinking about. At the time this happened I did not appreciate how dangerous a situation it was and it is only on reflection, when I consider the possible outcomes, that it really hits home.

It was a few years later, when I was developing part of the basement that another incident happened which was rather painful for me and could have possibly been a lot more serious than it actually turned out. I was doing some electrical wiring in the ceiling and I was standing on the seat of an armchair so that I could reach the area where I was working. Although I could reach the spot okay, I found that after a few minutes my arms began to ache, as I was extending them too much. To resolve this problem, I needed to be closer to the ceiling, so I decided to step up onto the arm of the armchair which had arms that were about 8 inches wide and provided plenty of room for me to stand on. Of course I must not have been giving much thought to what I was doing because as I transferred my weight onto the arm of the chair, it suddenly tipped over. As it tipped I fell towards the other arm of the chair and my left side met it coming up. The impact actually broke the wooden structure of the arm. I was in considerable pain as might be expected, and our son Michael, who was assisting me at the time, said "Would you like a cup of tea, Dad?" to try to take my mind off my suffering. [The 'magic' cup of tea is supposed to solve all problems].

To make sure that I had not broken any ribs I had Lilian drive me to the Hospital Emergency. When I was finally attended to, I was sent for x-rays of my left chest area. As I was being asked to change position for the different areas to be x-rayed I was wincing with pain and the Doctor in attendance said, "If you think this is bad now, just wait, it's going to get <u>a lot</u> worse". The x-rays did not show any broken bones nor any severe fractures, although I felt that there must have been some 'hair-line fractures' even though the technicians said they couldn't see any.

When the Doctor made that comment about the pain I was going through he knew what he was talking about. I was actually disabled for about a week and could hardly move at all without inflicting some terrible pain on myself. I was clad in my pyjamas and dressing gown for the whole time and I couldn't stand the pain every time I moved. My son Andrew thought it was great fun to tell me funny stories in order to make me laugh, and when I did laugh there were also tears of pain running down my face at the same time. Overall, I was thankful that my injuries were not much worse, which they might well have been and it seemed that Lady Luck may have smiled on me yet again. My neck could have been broken if I had fallen more awkwardly. This was just another mishap when my body took a bit of a beating, and is not included in my lucky escapes from death.

As the years went by, I finally settled into a reasonably well paid job as an Insurance Agent, [the harder one worked the more lucrative it could be]. We managed to take trips back home to England every two or three years and luckily we had relatives that we could stay with while we were there. This helped quite a bit in keeping the overall costs down. At first we would stay with our parents and later, after they had passed away, other relatives would step into the breach. Pauline, Lil's sister, and her husband Brian put us up a number of times, and Sheila, another of Lil's sisters, and her husband Ron also accommodated us a few times. Whenever we visited my brother Charlie and his wife Mary just outside York, they would kindly let us stay with them. We used to take some pleasant side trips around Britain, usually with various family members, and we were often told by our relatives that they would never have visited most of these places if we hadn't been over and arranged the trips. We ourselves had never been to Scotland until after we had emigrated to Canada and had come back to England [Britain] for a holiday.

From time to time we used to get relatives visiting us for a holiday, in Canada. On one occasion we actually had eleven people [including ourselves] staying at our house at the same time. We used to show them around and sometimes take trips with them to areas of interest, mostly around Alberta or B.C. and I remember a couple of trips into the States. It was on one of our sightseeing trips in

Alberta, I think it was during the early eighties, that I had my next lucky escape from death. We were on a day trip to Drumheller and had started out fairly early to make a long day of it. It was in the height of summer and we were in for a hot day. Because there were nine of us altogether, we travelled in two cars. There were five in my car and four in our other car which Lil was driving. When we reached Drumheller there was a 'pancake breakfast' still going on, so we gladly joined in and enjoyed some of the goodies. Our company was quite surprised by the fact that we did not have to pay for it. It was their first experience of a stampede breakfast and they thought it was just great. We spent the day visiting tourist attractions with intermittent spells of eating and eventually finishing off with dinner at a local restaurant, before heading back to Calgary. The timing for our drive back could have been better. The sun was getting low in the clear sky and we were heading straight towards it, which made the driving a bit awkward to say the least. However, as we proceeded on our journey, we took the road to Beiseker which was about forty miles straight West with only one lane in each direction and no hard shoulders. The speed limit on this road was 60 m.p.h. I was driving in front, at the speed limit, with Lil following behind. At this point I would like to mention that we had a sort of family rule for when we were out driving any distance. Whoever was sitting in the front passenger seat would have to be sure to stay awake so that he or she could make certain that the driver did not fall asleep at the wheel. Usually it was me who would be driving and Lilian who would be in the front with me. She was most diligent in staying awake on any trip and often had to get my attention when it looked like I might be nodding off and this rule worked very well to keep us all safe and sound. However, on this particular trip out, the rule was overlooked because Lil and I were in separate cars, which is why what I am about to relate was allowed to happen.

Every one in my car had 'flaked out' as we had had a very tiring day so it could have been expected that this might happen. I had decided that I would <u>not</u> fall asleep like the rest of my passengers had done, so I turned up the radio and wound down the drivers window in an effort to help me keep alert. The next thing I remember was being jolted awake as the front wheel of the car had bumped off the tarmac and back on again. Apparently [as I was told later] I had been weaving back and forth into the oncoming lane and they, in the car behind, had been unable to get my attention by blasting the horn. If I had encountered an oncoming car as I veered into the other lane we would have collided at a closing speed of at least 120 m.p.h. and God only knows what carnage would have been caused. I was extremely fortunate that the car didn't roll into the ditch when the front wheel left the road. For some reason there had been a short stretch of additional tarmac, about two feet wide, laid along the edge of the road that was approximately 50 to 100 feet in length, and about two or three inches lower than the road surface. This was to bolster a weak part of the edge of the road. It was at this precise spot that the wheel 'decided' to drop off the road's edge. Anywhere else along that road and we would have gone into the ditch and rolled at 60 M.P.H. and I don't think any of us in my car would have stood a chance for survival. This was at a time when there was no by-law about wearing seat belts, and nobody in my car had had them fastened. I consider myself to have been extremely lucky that this situation resolved itself the way it did. It still gives me the shivers every time I bring it to mind. I don't know how long I was asleep for, but it only takes a second for things to go all horribly wrong. Many lives could have been lost that day, not only for those of us who were in our party, but those of the people who might have been unfortunate enough to have collided with us during one of my veerings into the oncoming lane. When I realised what had just happened I was literally shocked into staying awake for the rest of the drive home, although we had to wait until we reached Beiseker before we could pull in to refresh ourselves, because of the absence of any hard shoulder on the road we were travelling on. This was definitely my <u>sixth</u> lucky escape from death. Of course, my passengers could also count this episode as a lucky escape from death, if they had been keeping any score in the matter.

As the years went by, our three kids, Andrew, Michael, and Alison all did exceedingly well at school and they all managed to graduate, with honours, from the University of Calgary. If we had not emigrated to Canada I don't know if they would have attained this higher level of education as there definitely seemed to be more opportunities for students to attend university here than there were in Britain. All three of them were very diligent in obtaining summer jobs and putting a lot of their pay aside towards university fees. They all happened to win various scholarships through high school and university which enabled them to pay there their own way and it really helped us with our family finances. The fact that we lived quite close to Calgary University enabled them all to live at home for the duration and they did not have the hassle of having to find accommodation. As I have mentioned before, Lilian and I were very proud of all three of them and they all now realise that their perseverance throughout their school years has helped them considerably in obtaining good employment and the fact that they had been sensible and thrifty with any monies which came their way has, in its turn, also helped them in setting up their own homes.

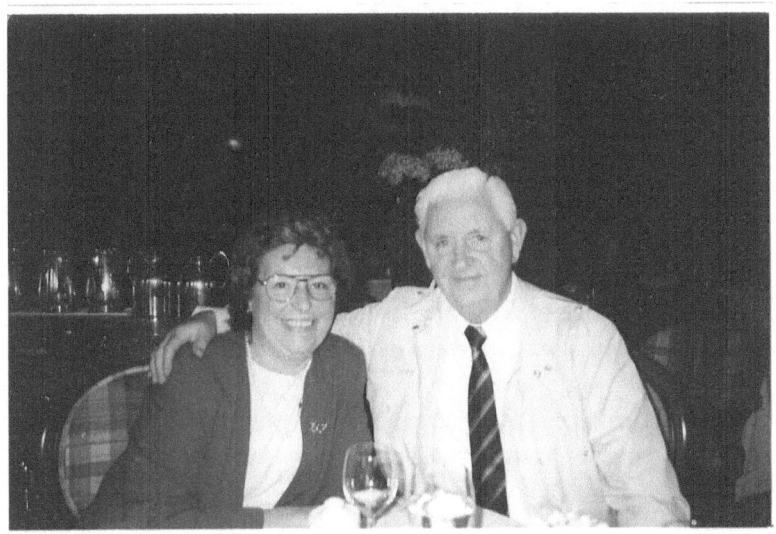

A photo of myself [The Author] and Lilian my wife enjoying a meal out in Aug. 1998.

This was on the occasion when Lil. had been selected as 'Secretary of the week' by a local radio station in Calgary and the meal for two was included in the award.

8

It was about ten or eleven years after the Drumheller trip, when I had just had my 59th birthday, that I finally pulled the plug on working for a living. My company had offered me the chance to have a severance package to take early retirement, so after discussing our financial position with Lil, we decided [jointly] that it would be a good idea to accept the offer, and it gave the company the opportunity to install a person who was about twenty five years younger. [It seems that youth is preferable to experience]. We had been fairly frugal over the years despite all our trips over to England etc. and there were sufficient funds available for us to survive, and still have a decent vacation each year. This situation was largely due to Lil's excellent money management over the years. Lil decided to carry on working in the part time job she had as a Legal Secretary, although she was always able to get the time off that we needed for a lengthy holiday in England, albeit without pay. To supplement our income we both took our Canada pension three years early, [at age 62], at a reduced rate. I am so thankful that I did take the early retirement, because it enabled Lil and I to spend a lot more time together, but we never suspected that a couple of years later, fate was about to deal us a couple of terribly <u>cruel</u> blows.

Following a routine medical check-up, Lil was diagnosed with an advanced stage of colon cancer which meant that she had to have the whole of her colon removed in December 1999, followed by chemotherapy. The prognosis by the oncologist was that the cancer had spread to other organs and Lil had only 36 months left and it was such a devastating shock. However, Lil recovered quite well after the operation and the chemotherapy sessions did not seem too upsetting. So much so that she was strong enough for us to take our planned trip to England in August 2000. We had also planned for a side trip of a week in Nice on the French Riviera. Our daughter Alison had decided to join us on this vacation, although she would have to return to Canada a bit sooner than ourselves, after we returned to England from our week in Nice [the curse of the working classes].

It was on this particular holiday that I was to have my next confrontation with the 'grim reaper'. Our week in France was going quite nicely when certain things happened which I did not associate with any impending problem. We were hurrying along the road one morning to catch a bus to Monte Carlo when I experienced a rather dry feeling in my chest, just to the right of my sternum [chest bone]. I put it down to the heat and proceeded to drink from the water bottle which I was carrying. As we reached the bus depot and boarded the bus, the dry feeling subsided and I thought no more about it.

At this point I would like to mention that there was a taxi strike on in Nice, the reason for which we were not aware of, and a lot of taxis were blockading the airport, obviously to cause as much disruption as possible for travellers and hence get the maximum publicity to further their cause. When it was time for us to leave for the airport for our return trip to Manchester to continue with the rest of our England trip, we could not get a taxi, because they were all already at the airport doing their blockading. We were told by the hotel staff that there was an Airport bus which we could catch at a stop about three blocks away from the hotel. As we struggled up the road with our luggage, I was carrying four bags; one in each hand and one under each arm. Again I experienced that dryness feeling in my chest and once again put it down to the heat. After all, we were on the French Riviera, so it must be the heat. Once again I used the water bottle after we had reached the bus stop and put the bags down, and again the dryness feeling went away and we forgot all about it. While we were waiting at the bus stop we noticed that we were right outside the Cardiac Centre Building and we were actually joking about being in the right place should we have any problems. Upon reflection, it was all rather ironic in view of what was about to happen a couple of days later when we were back in England.

The bus was due at 12.25 p.m. so we arrived at the bus stop about ten minutes earlier, to be sure not to miss it, but it didn't arrive until 1.30 p.m. which had left us standing for over an hour at the hottest time of the day. Not only was the bus very late, but it was also very crowded, as a lot of other travellers had had the same idea due to the taxi strike. They also were carrying their luggage. Anyway, we managed to squeeze ourselves onto the bus and it headed towards the airport. It stopped at a few more hotels which were en route and picked up even more passengers. We were so tightly packed in that it looked like a bus from some third world country.

When we got to Nice Airport the driver had to drop us off at quite some distance from the terminal as the taxi blockade was in place and this was the only spot that the bus could turn around to head back to town. However, I managed to find a luggage cart and loaded our bags onto it and proceeded towards the terminal. Because of all the delays, when we arrived at the check-in desk, we were only just in time to catch our flight to Manchester.

As I had pre-ordered a rental car at Manchester airport, as soon as we arrived there, we headed for the rental desk and attempted to organise it. Each time the agent punched in my credit card number it came up as cancelled. It transpired that a couple of years earlier, while we were on holiday in England, Lilian had lost a credit card receipt which had the full card number on it, so she promptly phoned and cancelled her card as a precautionary measure. It was replaced a short while later, but somehow the Mastercard people in <u>England</u> were showing both our cards as cancelled, [Lil's card was a secondary one to mine and they both had different numbers.] This confusion led to several phone calls to MasterCard in <u>Canada</u> and each time we spoke I was told that my card was in good standing. When the rental agent called the MasterCard people in England they kept telling him that my card showed up on their system as cancelled. Despite several attempts to try and get the credit card people in Canada to converse with their counterparts in England, neither one would speak with the other, which left us with a very frustrating situation. Just by chance the Canadian bank called me back and asked me if the agent had actually 'swiped' the card through his machine, but as his machine was damaged he had been punching the number in when he was connected to the MasterCard office in England. Luckily there was another office for the same rental company in one of the other terminals at Manchester airport, so we loaded up the car with the luggage and ourselves and the agent, and drove over to the other office. The agent took the card and 'swiped' it through their machine and—Problem solved. All this rigmarole had taken up the best part of two hours and the strain of all the arguing did not bode well with my health as will be seen shortly. The credit card was the only way I could pay for the rental, which is why the episode was so upsetting. It was either that or put down about 800 pounds cash, which we didn't have available.

At this time in England, there what was known as a PETROL STRIKE taking place, the reason for which we never did find out. What was happening was that all the refineries in Britain were being blockaded and none of the petrol tankers were being allowed through to pick up supplies. Hence all the petrol stations across Britain were running dry. The people who were doing the blockading were condescending enough to let some emergency supplies through, which were intended for, Doctors, Police, Ambulances, and Fire Departments and associated employees only. Occasionally a petrol station would have some supplies left over, which gave rise to queues of cars of 50 or more in both directions approaching the particular station. People would be waiting for lengthy periods and, to avoid any 'cheating' in line, police were brought in to direct them.

My brother Charlie had come down by train from York, where he lived, to visit with us at Runcorn, where we were staying with other relatives. The four of us [Lilian and I, Charlie, and Alison] had planned for a day out to Conway in North Wales, where Charlie and I were evacuated during the War, which was about a hundred miles or so from where we were staying. I estimated that the trip both ways plus extra running around while we were there would come to nearly 300 miles. The date was 9/11/2000, just one year to the day prior to the New York towers disaster. Alison had come to the end of her stay, and was due to return to Canada the next day, and I had only a half tank of petrol. It was agreed that we would not go for the planned run out into North Wales, but would keep the petrol to take her to Manchester Airport the following day, which would be around 25 miles each way, and after that we would just have to take our chances in getting further supplies of petrol. As some bus depots used to keep reserves of fuel on site, it was probable that some buses would still be running and our relatives, Sheila, Lil's sister, and her husband Ron, [in whose house we were staying] told us that there was a bus stop at the end of their road where one could catch a bus which went into Manchester Airport.

To recap for a moment, when Alison had flown over from Calgary she had gone to Heathrow Airport and had an extra return ticket to Manchester. However, she had planned to visit relatives in the London area and then come up to Runcorn by train, which she did, and in doing so did not use the first half of the return ticket to Manchester. This meant that she would not be allowed to use the return half back to London. [Apparently there is some weird condition attached to the return half which cancels it, if the first half is not used.]

Lilian and I had come over to England a bit later than Alison and she was to meet us at Manchester airport, where the three of us were to catch the flight to Nice from Manchester, later in the afternoon.

While we were at the airport, we had a couple of hours or so to wait for our flight to Nice, so, the three of us took the opportunity to confer with a representative of the airline that Alison would be using for her return flight to London. The agent we spoke to was most helpful, and, to cut a long story short, we managed to have the return half of her ticket reinstated.

Now back to 9/11/2000. As an alternate plan, we decided to try taking the bus to the airport for a dry run, and see if it would be more prudent to go by bus the next day when Alison would be leaving, rather than going by car and in doing so save the petrol. Of course, we wouldn't know for sure if the bus would be running the next day or not. Anyway, it would be a little outing for us, and we could always fall back on using the rental car, if necessary, the next day. Just before we were about to leave to catch the bus, I went and moved the car from the curbside and put it on the driveway. As I got out of the car to go back into the house, I once again felt that dry feeling on the right side of my chest. I went into the house and suddenly I broke out in a very heavy sweat, all over my chest. So much so that I needed a towel to wipe it up. It was Ron, my brother-in-law, who recognised the symptoms and told Sheila to call an ambulance. It only took about five minutes for the ambulance to arrive, as they were cruising in the area. When the paramedics came in, I felt quite normal, and also felt like a bit of a fraud wasting the ambulance's time. However, when my symptoms had been described to them they insisted that I should be taken to the hospital to be checked out. They were wheeling me out in a chair and as we passed the car, I said "Don't scratch the car, it's a rental". After they had lifted me into the back of the ambulance, I was asked to sit on the bed and then to lie down while they asked me some personal details. They got as far as my name and date of birth, when I suddenly felt myself fading away and I just said to the paramedic "I'm going" and then everything just went black. [I found out later that I had undergone a cardiac arrest]. The next thing I remember I had come 'to' on the gurney being wheeled into the hospital at Halton, by Runcorn, and the paramedic was telling the Doctor in the 'Emergency', "I have 'shocked' him three times". Believe me, that was of course a fourth shock, when I realised that it was me that they were talking about. I was incredibly lucky that it had all happened while I was in the ambulance.

This occasion was indeed the most serious of all my lucky escapes from death, [My <u>seventh</u>] and whenever anybody mentions the date of 9/11, it has a special significance for myself and my family. I have heard that 50% of people who have a heart attack don't make it past the first one, and if we had gone out for our drive as planned, it would have happened while we were on the motorway and who knows what kind of disaster might have been caused by the inevitable crash or pile up that would have ensued, as I was the one who would have been driving. It is frightening to think of how many lives might have been lost. Even if I had had time to pull over, which I doubt, I know that I would not have made it because the ambulance would not have reached us in time. We have the PETROL STRIKE to thank, as that was the reason we didn't want to use up the limited supply of petrol that we had and it caused us to change our plans. Several lives, besides my own, might have been spared that day because of the unusual circumstances.

Because of what had happened, Alison did not take her flight back the next day but stayed to visit with me in Hospital for the next week or so, until the doctors had considered me to be out of immediate danger.

After I was admitted to the Hospital Emergency, the staff managed to get me stabilised for the moment, but over the course of the next two days I had two more Cardiac Arrests which certainly kept the staff hopping. Lilian, my wife, was told by the cardiologist that if I had any more attacks that they would have to send me by ambulance to Broadgreen Hospital in Liverpool, which had a proper cardiac unit and had all the sophisticated equipment to deal with such a situation, as Halton Hospital [the one I was in] was only a small Rural Hospital and they were not as well equipped. However, she was also told that it was possible that I might not survive the journey. That's how serious it was. Broadgreen Hospital was about eleven miles away by road.

As luck would have it they managed to keep me stabilised and after four days in Emergency I was moved to a regular ward where I spent another seven days, after which I was discharged. It was in this ward that I met Mike Crowe who was having heart valve trouble and we kept each others spirits up by telling jokes etc and we have kept in touch since then. I always visit with Mike and his wife Chris and their two daughters whenever I go for a holiday in England, and I am always made to feel very welcome.

I was advised by the cardiologist that I should not fly back to Canada for at least six weeks. I couldn't do much else as the Air Canada doctors would not let me fly back without an 'all clear' from the cardiologist. Hence, Lil and I decided to stay in a hotel as we did not want to infringe upon Lil's sister, Sheila and her husband Ron, in whose house we had been staying, as we were expected to be there for six weeks before returning home to Canada. We were staying in a hotel in a small town called Frodsham which was only about two or three miles from Halton Hospital. Being this close to the Hospital made me feel a bit more secure. With regards to the rental vehicle, I had put Ron on as an additional driver at the time we picked up the car, so while I was in Hospital he kindly returned the vehicle to the Manchester Airport office, which was about three weeks earlier than the original contract. When I was discharged I was, of course, not allowed to do any driving.

There is a little story I would like to tell about our stay in Frodsham for the six weeks, which really emphasises how 'lucky' I really was. Across the main street from our hotel in Frodsham there was a small general store which also housed a Post Office. One day, the man who owned the store happened to notice a youth who was trying to steal some pens. As the youth left the store the owner took chase after him, running down the road, but the boy managed to jump on a bus that was just about to leave and so escaped. The store owner walked back to the store and as soon as he got to it he collapsed with a heart attack. The ambulance was called but when it arrived it was already too late for them to save him. It made me so thankful that I had been 'lucky' enough to survive. It makes one realise just how suddenly things can take a turn for the worse.

Whilst we were spending our time in the hotel in Frodsham I had to attend a clinic each week which was for checking my blood, as I was on blood thinning tablets. If it wasn't at the thinness it was supposed to be, the dosage of the tablets [Warfarin] would be adjusted, and eventually it would be stabilised at the right level. I also had to attend a local Doctor each week for him to check me over. I supposed that if my health was in any danger I might have had my movements restricted and maybe the 'no flying' period extended. I used to get a little exercise each day by walking up and down the street in front of the Hotel and by climbing to the first floor, [two or three times] up the long staircase, which was in the lobby of the Hotel.

Our long time good friends Sheila and Paul Winter [whom we had known ever since we moved into our house in Crosfield Road in Prescot, all those years ago] would come over to the Hotel and take us out for a drive each Wednesday. This was quite a pleasant and welcome diversion which also helped to break the monotony. The one slight drawback that I didn't mention to anyone at the time was that I tended to get a little panicky the further we moved away from the Hospital. It felt like I was stretching the 'lifeline', but I didn't want to spoil the outings or upset our friends. They had taken the time to plan a different trip out each week and Lil and I were so very grateful to them for being so thoughtful and looking after us. We all enjoyed ourselves on each of these outings and it also gave us the chance to have a good old 'chin-wag' and everything worked out well in the end.

I would also like to mention that Sheila and Paul, along with their three young boys, also lived in Crosfield Road, [even before we moved there], and we were very good friends with them. Each time we went over to England for a holiday, the Winter family were always on the top of our list of friends with whom we were going to visit. They had, of course, moved to Widnes shortly after we had emigrated to Canada.

9

When we finally were given the 'O.K.' to return to Canada, I was told that I would have to have an oxygen supply on the plane, in a sufficient amount to cover the six hours flight to Toronto, and similarly to cover the four hours flight from Toronto to Calgary. According to the cardiologist's calculations, we would need six cylinders on the first flight and four on the second. There had to be enough supply to cover the worst scenario [which would need one cylinder per hour]. As things turned out I did not need to use the oxygen at all. [thank goodness]. Although I didn't feel too bad, I was instructed to use a wheelchair at each of the three Airports, as Air Canada did not want to be liable for any mishap that might happen through my not using one. I must admit it felt strange, but I complied with their instructions on the premise that 'It's better to be safe than sorry'.

When we finally got back to Calgary at the end of Oct. 2000, I obtained a referral from my G.P. to see a cardiologist, [22 nd Dec. 2000.] The waiting period was just about two months. Lilian had appointments on a weekly basis for more chemotherapy treatments, which turned out to be somewhat stronger than her previous ones, and meant that she would lose her hair in the process. She carried on with no complaints and I think she was worrying more about me than herself, but that was Lil's nature, always concerned for others more than herself.

It was just one day prior to my cardiologist appointment when I experienced that dryness feeling in my chest again, so we went straight over to my Doctor's office and he saw me right away. After a quick cursory examination he said to Lilian, "I want you to take him to the emergency RIGHT NOW". He gave us a note to give to the Doctor at the Hospital in which he suggested an angiogram might be needed. As my condition was so serious, we went back home and called an ambulance. We were not going to take the chance of my going into 'Cardiac Arrest' again, before anyone could see me in emergency. [At that time people were having to wait up to 18 hours before being attended to] If it happened again as it did in England it would be more prudent to have the paramedics on hand in the ambulance. The paramedics did an E.K.G. on me while en route and had it ready to give to the doctor at the hospital. Although I was being attended to in emergency by nurses and a Doctor, I did not get to see a Cardiologist for about 18 hours. The Doctor who was looking after me while we were waiting for the cardiologist was originally from Korea, and he told me that in Korea if one needed to see a cardiologist he could see one immediately. As it was just prior to Christmas 2000, [21 st Dec] it was fortunate that there were staff available to perform an angiogram followed by an angioplasty [stent]. My diagnosis was that I had one artery blocked 100%, [L.A.D.] which they could not get into and one artery blocked 90% [D.1.] which was the one that was stented and a certain amount of damage had been sustained to the heart muscle by the 3 cardiac arrests which happened in England.

I was released from Hospital after a few days when it was determined that I was out of danger and I was advised to avoid large meals and to cut down on fat and salt and to try and walk 2 kilometres a day. All this was going on while Lil was undergoing her treatments and for the next two years we sort of looked after each other. I am so thankful that I was able to take care of Lil and shudder to think what might have happened to her if I had not been there to take her to her appointments and prepare her some food when she needed it, etc. Then Lil had a bit of a setback and further surgery was needed. This time she had to have a hysterectomy and unfortunately her health took a downturn after it was done. This was in May 2002. A couple of months later she started a further course of chemotherapy, which I reckoned was a bit too soon after her surgery and it only seemed to worsen her condition and sadly she slowly deteriorated until she finally passed away in February 2003. This was by far the saddest period of my life and I still feel that I will never get over her loss.

After you lose someone like this you tend to think of things that you now regret. Over the years Lil and I had travelled to many places together across Europe, America and Britain, but there was one particular place that Lil had always wanted to visit and that was Egypt, so she could see the pyramids first hand. There was so much violence going on in the Middle East that it was I who was so reluctant to go there. There had been all kinds of attacks on tourists in the area so I put my foot down and would not go there as I considered it to be unsafe. Now, of course, I deeply regret that we didn't go there to fulfil Lil's lifelong dream, and all of a sudden it's too late to do anything about it.

The biggest regret of all is the fact that Lil never got to see any of our three children married. It's every Mothers dream to see their off-springs married and settled down and even have a hand in organising their weddings. Andrew and Vivianne eloped to Jamaica several years earlier [1992] and neither of us got to see them hitched. They are currently raising two daughters; Julia and Victoria who are growing into two fine young ladies. Michael and Tamiko were married in Calgary [Sept. 2003] just seven months after Lil had passed away. Alison and Russ were married, also in Calgary, almost a year later [Aug. 2004]. These were two very happy occasions, which everybody thoroughly enjoyed, but I could not help also feeling a deep sadness because Lilian was not able to be there, and I know Mike, and Alison also felt her absence very much.

I miss Lil so much and for so many reasons that whenever I think about her I always remember the words from a song by Joni Mitchell [Big Yellow Taxi] which read, 'You don't know what you've got 'till it's gone' and believe me that is so very true. I often quote those words to couples whenever I hear them fighting or squabbling, mostly over stupid unimportant things, as people tend to do.

It was April 1st 2004 when, one morning, [now living on my own] I once again experienced a bout of heavy sweating. As I was used to doing a spell on the treadmill each morning, I debated with myself whether to do the treadmill as usual or send for an Ambulance. Not to take any chances I called for an Ambulance, telling the operator that I thought I was having another Heart Attack. The Ambulance arrived in a short space of time, and the paramedics prepped me and whisked me off again to Calgary Foothills Hospital Emergency. On this occasion I was taken almost immediately to surgery where an Angiogram was performed and another artery on my heart [R.C.A.] was found to be about 90% blocked and it was stented right away. I can only hazard a guess as to what might have happened had I not called for the ambulance when I did.

I recovered very quickly and was able to return home the next day. Things seemed to be going okay for the next few days when, suddenly, I experienced a problem with my stomach and bowel. It was known as a 'Paralysed Ileus' [I think I have the term correct]. Part of the small intestine shuts down with the result that nothing can go through one's system. Fortunately, when it happened, my daughter Alison was staying over because I was not feeling well. That night, I collapsed in the bathroom due to dehydration, and she phoned for an ambulance. Of course the Fire Department also sent a truck in case there was any rescuing to be done, which there was. When I had fallen in the bathroom, I was slumped against the door and Alison could not open it, and a fireman had to get me to shuffle away from the door so that he could get inside and help me to my feet. If Alison had not been there, I don't know what would have happened as I was completely "out of it". <u>Luckily</u> she was and I was taken care of by the paramedics and once again I was taken into Hospital. I spent the next day in the emergency ward. They said I was fine and released me, and my son Michael suggested I stay at their house for a couple of days. However, that night, the pressure in my stomach continued to build causing me to be severely sick. They called for an ambulance and I was taken into a different Hospital where I spent a further eleven days with a tube through my nose and into my stomach to keep draining it to avoid any build up. Apparently, this is a condition which is not uncommon, and can happen to patients about five days after surgery, and eventually rights itself in due course. Not a pleasant experience, I assure you. I lost weight during that hospital stay to the tune of 20 lbs, which I think I have put back on again since then. [Ah well.]

Since then my condition has been virtually stable and I have been following my Cardiologist's advice, along with taking a host of medications, and I try to get some moderate exercise each day, [usually walking]. I still am bothered by the cold air or wind and I cannot walk outside if the temperature is below about plus 15 degrees C., and because of this, most of my walking is done in shopping malls, although I have the treadmill at home and try to do some walking on it every day. I decided to try to walk 2 miles per day and as I have now been doing this for 7 years I have come up with an interesting statistic; By my calculations I have walked about 5,100 miles in that time and as Mount Everest is approx. 5.1 miles high, I have walked 1,000 times its height, [and still walking]. I hope this doesn't mean that I will reach Heaven any time soon!

To add 'insult to injury' as they say, in March 2006, I experienced some severely painful attacks across my midriff and was yet again transported to Calgary Foothills hospital by ambulance. After undergoing several tests over the next six days to find out the cause of the attacks, it was finally diagnosed as a gall bladder problem. My gall bladder was removed [30 March 2006] and after another 6 days I was discharged. I have recovered quite well from this latest 'situation' and I was also surprised when I was told that it would not be necessary to make any changes to my diet. This episode is not being added to the list of my escapes from death.

I tend to rely heavily on my car to get me around but, if I continue to behave myself and obey all the rules, I hope to live many more years, despite having all the restrictions, and I aim to stave off the 'cashing in' of my "Eighth and Ninth lives" for as long as possible.

On reflection, I would say that throughout my life so far I have been rather <u>unfortunate</u> in encountering so many dangerous situations which could have caused me to be maimed or disabled in some way or even resulted in my death. At the same time I must say that I have also been <u>extremely</u> <u>lucky</u> to have come through all that has happened, despite currently being left somewhat less than 100% fit and able.

Even though up to now I have beaten DEATH <u>at least seven</u> times, it doesn't matter how many more times I can beat the odds, because eventually, …

'DEATH' only needs to win ONCE!

978-0-595-49844-4
0-595-49844-2